The COPD Solution

the **COPD SOLUTION**

*A Proven 10-Week Program
for Living and Breathing Better
with Chronic Lung Disease*

Dawn Lesley Fielding, BS, RCP, AE-C

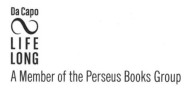

Da Capo
LIFE
LONG
A Member of the Perseus Books Group

Copyright © 2015 by Dawn Lesley Fielding
Photos courtesy of the author

Designed by Timm Bryson
Set in 11.5 point Minion Pro by the Perseus Books Group

Cataloging-in-Publication data for this book is available from the Library of Congress.

First Da Capo Press edition 2015
ISBN: 978-0-7382-1825-0 (paperback)
ISBN: 978-0-7382-1826-7 (e-book)

Published by Da Capo Press
A Member of the Perseus Books Group
www.dacapopress.com

Note: The information in this book is true and complete to the best of our knowledge. This book is intended only as an informative guide for those wishing to know more about health issues. In no way is this book intended to replace, countermand, or conflict with the advice given to you by your own physician. The ultimate decision concerning care should be made between you and your doctor. We strongly recommend you follow his or her advice. Information in this book is general and is offered with no guarantees on the part of the authors or Da Capo Press. The authors and publisher disclaim all liability in connection with the use of this book.

Da Capo Press books are available at special discounts for bulk purchases in the U.S. by corporations, institutions, and other organizations. For more information, please contact the Special Markets Department at the Perseus Books Group, 2300 Chestnut Street, Suite 200, Philadelphia, PA, 19103, or call (800) 810-4145, ext. 5000, or e-mail special .markets@perseusbooks.com.

10 9 8 7 6 5 4 3 2 1

For sweet Jude, Linda, Jan, Bob, Charlie, and so many more who continue to press on, smiling through breathlessness, anxiety, and so much more to discover strength and find beauty in every day, thank you. You continue to inspire me to sing the beautiful song of life. Breathe easy, my dear friends.

Finish each day and be done with it. You have done what you could. Some blunders and absurdities no doubt crept in; forget them as soon as you can. Tomorrow is a new day; begin it well and serenely and with too high a spirit to be cumbered with your old nonsense.

—RALPH WALDO EMERSON

CONTENTS

Contents

FOREWORD

There is sometimes a moment when the universe aligns—a moment that is explosive, large, loud, invisible, and silent all at the same time—when time seems to stop, and a purpose is born. For everyone who experiences this, it may be different. For me, it started with a fire in my chest, a burning that spread throughout my body, all the way to my fingertips and toes. My head was on fire, too, and I think it might have actually physically enlarged from the impact. I knew what I wanted to do. I knew where I was needed. And I readied myself for the journey.

With the numbers of those afflicted rapidly climbing the charts, the problems of chronic obstructive pulmonary disease (COPD) are quickly becoming a worldwide concern. In order to relieve the pain and suffering its victims experience, and out of an incredible lack of resources and tools available for those who proudly wear its badge, *The COPD Solution* was born.

I am compelled to raise awareness of the impact of this disease—and I want anyone who suffers from this illness to know that there is hope, there is a strategy, you can gain ability, and you can be given tools to do so much more than merely survive.

Treating COPD has become my mission. I am here to serve you. I hope you find in the pages of this book what my experience, determination, love, hope, and practice have shown so many others. I hope you begin to *live and thrive* rather than simply be *alive*. I am so happy to be your therapist!

Best wishes and happy breathing,
DLF

PART 1

LIVING WITH CHRONIC LUNG DISEASE

CHAPTER ONE

When You Can't Breathe, Nothing Else Matters

When you own your own breath, nobody can steal your peace.

—AUTHOR UNKNOWN

I'd like to introduce you to Linda. Linda is 64 years old, 5'4" tall, and weighs 155 pounds. She has been diagnosed with chronic obstructive pulmonary disease (COPD), an umbrella term commonly used for the combination of any two of the following chronic lung diseases: emphysema, chronic bronchitis, or asthma. Linda was diagnosed four years ago. A recent test of her breathing function placed her in the Stage III category for COPD—that is, severe. This is the story of the first time I met her. Her story may remind you of yourself or someone you love.

I had already started my assessment of her before we were even close enough to speak. Linda has short, brown hair. It has been cut, I am assuming, for easy upkeep (most patients with her condition struggle to perform tasks above the waist). She has dark, deep-set eyes, and wears no makeup. Although she is Caucasian, her skin has a slight natural tan. She has a few more wrinkles than do most people her age. Her movements are very slow and deliberate, and she kind of shuffles when she walks, as if it is an effort to lift her feet.

Linda is quiet and concentrated. She looks focused as she approaches me. Her breathing is labored, and I can hear her wheezing and see the retractions in her neck as the gap between us shrinks. Her mouth is drawn slightly open, her lips curling inward just a bit. It pronounces her cheekbones in a unique way. I have seen many patients in her condition hold their mouth this same way in an effort to "catch more air." I make a mental note to review proper breathing techniques with her as soon as possible.

Looking out the window, I notice the silver car she exited is parked in the first handicapped spot by the door—that's only 60 feet or so from where she is, but it has taken a great amount of effort to get here. It's safe to assume she will need a rest soon, and that she has to rest countless times throughout her day.

Finally, she reaches the door to my office. "Hi Linda, I'm Dawn," I say, and motion toward a chair in my lobby. She quickly accepts the invitation to sit but can't quite thank me—not yet. She's too breathless to speak. After a few minutes of silence, except for the hissing of the portable oxygen tank she has brought along with her, she thanks me for my patience and indicates that she is now able to proceed. As I talk to her, and having reviewed her pulmonary function paperwork from her physician, I mentally catalog my list of her signs and symptoms. They include:

Breathing Symptoms

- Severe dyspnea (shortness of breath). Even resting, she has extreme difficulty completing a short sentence in one breath.
- Wheezing
- Productive cough
- Retractions (a sucking in of the skin around the bones in the chest cavity during inhalation)
- Air trapping (when air gets trapped in the lungs due to a decrease in lung function)

- Hypoxia (low oxygen levels)
- Lung function testing shows a decreased FEV1 (amount of air you can exhale in one second) that is 28% of the expected volume

Other Physical Symptoms

- Extreme fatigue
- Severely reduced physical activity
- Muscle weakness. She is shaking, and, although her oxygen tank is on wheels, her daughter rolls it in for her.
- Deconditioning (a condition in which there is a reduced functional capacity of the body due to chronic illness)
- Barrel chest (a widening of the chest cavity due to air trapping)
- Ankle swelling (indicative of heart problems)
- Digital clubbing, also called "drumstick fingers": An enlargement or bulging of the tip of the finger with a downward curvature of the nail, caused by chronic hypoxemia (low oxygen levels in the blood).
- Cyanosis (a bluish/gray color of the nail beds, caused by low oxygen)
- Nutritional deficiencies

Emotional Symptoms

- Extreme anxiety
- Depression and hopelessness

Exacerbations (Flare-Ups)

- Recent exacerbation of pneumonia
- A recent hospitalization
- 1–3 exacerbations yearly; at least one hospitalization yearly

Clearly, Linda has a lot to handle. I notice during the course of our conversation that she is on 4 liters of continuous oxygen via nasal cannula (a plastic tube device). She states that it is on that flow 24 hours per day. She also has hypoglycemia, also known as low blood sugar, and atherosclerosis, hardening of the arteries. She has a twenty-five-pack-year (at least one pack per year for twenty-five years) smoking history.

Her medications include a series of nebulizer treatments every four hours; oral medications for mucus control, anxiety, and depression; a combination inhaler to be used daily; another inhaler to be used twice daily; and yet another inhaler for emergencies. Her closet is full of oxygen tanks (I remind myself to talk to her about safety later), and her concentrator is located in her bedroom, where she feels she can properly control it at night.

Linda appears just as I expect a Stage III COPD patient to appear and presents a classic situation common to those with her diagnosis. She makes it known that she is very, very reluctant to meet with me. Her exact words are, "I am just going to die, anyway. I don't know why I am here."

When I hear this, I assure her first of all that she is not alone in feeling this way. But I ask, "Are you interested in staying if I promise that I can help you feel better?" This brings about a look of skepticism—a sideways glance of doubt. I invite her to stay, as I know, given the chance, I can change her mind. However, I can also tell she is going to be difficult to convince of this, so I ask her to list her concerns and tell me about herself. For now, I just listen.

During our conversation I find that she can only talk for a couple of sentences at a time, even with intermittent breaths carefully placed between words. Even then, she needs additional time to catch her breath. After these rests, the color returns to her lips and the tip of her nose, the gray fading back to pink. Also, her heart rate (I can see her pulse bounding in her neck) and respirations return to baseline when she rests. I wonder how much she would say if she weren't so limited. I wonder how much she used to smile and laugh when she spoke.

It takes a while, but I learn that Linda has three children. One of them, a daughter, passed away as a young adult. Her other daughter, who's brought her to the appointment, lives nearby, and her son lives in another state. She hasn't seen her son in three years because she can't go to him. The last time she tried, her oxygen tank ran out and she almost died. In addition, the presence of his dog makes it so she can't breathe. He doesn't have enough money to come and see her, and won't take the money she offers him to come. She recently gave her own dog away because the doctor said it would improve her breathing. She also gave her birds away last week. She cried about that.

Linda just had hardwood flooring put in her home, to prevent dust and dirt from building up in her carpet, and to avoid the need to vacuum, which she can't do any more. Her friend's son just moved into her basement in order to do household things for her, such as retrieve the mail, carry the laundry, and do the grocery shopping. She has someone come in to clean her house every other day, and her daughter and granddaughter bring her meals in or come over to fix them for her.

I learn that she used to like to gem hunt and spent a great amount of time doing so. She and her late husband, who died of COPD almost ten years ago, used to hunt, and make jewelry and furniture. She likes to quilt, but it's too difficult to do anymore. She hasn't done any of those things in a really long time, but she does still love to read. She used to enjoy watching her grandchildren play soccer. But most recently she doesn't have energy to do much of anything. In fact, making it to her doctor appointments is so much of an excursion she needs an entire day, or two sometimes, to recover.

She used to love to cook, but like so many other things, that is now too difficult to do. One of her greatest joys used to be fixing nice meals for her family. She used to be able to shower by herself, but now she can't. Her doctor has told her she is probably only going to live another year or so, and so she asks, why should she waste any of her time here?

Her daughter now interjects: "She used to be 'the life of the party.' Now, she just sits back and watches everything. She doesn't participate in life anymore. It's just not her. It's like this—" she motions her hands toward her mother "—is a shell of who my mom used to be. She's a ghost." Linda doesn't argue. Instead, she turns her eyes to the floor.

After a moment Linda speaks again, hinting toward some of her fears, but I get the impression she is scared to trust me with too much personal information, so I decide to move to the next step. The last thing I'm interested in doing is fostering any feelings of doubt.

"Can we try something called a six-minute walk test?" I ask. She has never heard of this before, but I'm not surprised, as most of my new patients haven't. This test is designed to establish a baseline for a care plan, determining what patients are capable of tolerating, and witnessing the degree of strength or weakness they are suffering from at any one particular moment. She looks at me suspiciously but doesn't answer. I wonder what is going through her head.

I smile at her and reassure her that I will walk with her, that she can rest whenever she needs to, and she only has to do what she can tolerate.

I set my timer, take Linda's hand and help her up, pick up her oxygen tank, and place an oximeter on her finger. An oximeter is a noninvasive device used to measure how much oxygen is in the blood, and, therefore, how much is available for the cells. And then, we begin to walk.

The circle we walk is 75 feet in diameter. We make it halfway around before she has to sit down and rest. I quickly lead her to the chair I had previously set aside for this occasion, and help her sit down. Her oxygen saturation levels, or sats, indicated by a number on the oximeter, started out at 94 percent on 4 liters of supplemental oxygen. Although she remained on her oxygen, that number is dropping now, and fast: 87 . . . 83 . . . 76 . . . 70 . . . 68. It finally stops.

Linda's anxiety is palpable. I can feel the crisis emanating from her. I look in her eyes to get her attention and focus on one not-so-simple thing: breathing. She puts her hand up, as if to stop time, or me, or everything, and closes her eyes as she tries to breathe. "Linda," I say gently, "look at me.

"In through your nose, then out through your mouth, like you're blowing out a candle." I say in a soft, calm voice. "This is the best way for you to recover, Linda. Do what I'm doing," I tell her. I demonstrate for her again. I inhale through my nose, and blow out through my pursed lips. In, and out. In, and out. "That's right. Smell the cake, blow out the candles. In, and out. In, and out." This goes on for one and a half minutes (which incidentally, can feel like an eternity). Again, her lips change from that familiar purple-blue to red, and the ashen coloring of her skin is replaced with a natural pink color. Her shaking is subsiding, and her heart rate, which had climbed to 148, is now returning to baseline.

I am not surprised to witness that she doesn't know how to perform pursed lip breathing. Although it is vital, most patients don't. We repeat the whole process as soon as she can walk again. We make it halfway around again, an echo of the same routine. This continues as the timer counted down the six minutes that it's been set for. Soon the timer rings, and her walk is complete. In total, she makes it around the circle almost four and a half times. Three hundred-thirty feet in six minutes' time, with four rests. Not at all that impressive.

After her walk and recovery, we talk more about her condition, her medications, her family, and how she feels about everything in general. Her depression is evident as I listen to her almost mourn her life. I explain what my program is, what we would do in it, what we would talk about, and how it would take place. She asks many questions, among others patients commonly ask, such as:

- What is COPD?
- Am I going to die? When?
- I know I need the oxygen, but why? How does it work?
- What exactly do my medications do?
- What will I get out of this program? How will I change? Will I change?
- Will I always be on oxygen?
- Will I ever get any better?
- How did I get this disease?
- What exactly has happened to my lungs?
- I. Can't. Breathe. Please help me. Can you really help me?
- Why did I do this to myself? I feel so guilty.

I explain a few of my expectations. I tell her I can help her, and teach her why she should "spend" some of her time here, and why it would not be a "waste" but actually, a really great investment. We also set goals. I tell her:

- I expect you to improve dramatically, if you do what I tell you to do. You will be surprised by how well you do.
- I will not hurt you. I promise.
- Did you know some foods make it more difficult to breathe? You will learn what to eat.
- You will get stronger.
- You will learn about your oxygen.
- You will learn about using energy.
- You will learn about your muscles and how your body uses oxygen.
- You will learn how to properly breathe.
- You will learn how you got this disease and what has happened inside your lungs so you can better understand what your struggle is.
- You will learn how to cough the right way. This will help with your mucus.
- You will learn to take your meds the correct way so they will help you the most.

And more important:
- You will improve so you can try to go see your son again.
- You will be able to do things, such as cook, on your own again. There are tricks I can teach you to do this.
- You will not only walk around this entire circle all at once (I motion to the circle she just walked that just about killed her), but you will actually walk much farther.
- You will do things you used to enjoy again.
- You will do these things *in only a few weeks' time.*
- You will learn why and how you can still live, not spend your time waiting to die.

Slowly, tears roll down her cheeks. Those same haunting eyes stare through me. She nods her head. Her daughter—who had pulled me aside earlier and held my hands as she begged me to save her mother, that I was her last hope—cries and mouths the words *thank you.*

Linda was scared, and my assumptions were correct—she was a difficult case. She was very, very sick. But, I had been successful in convincing her to try my program. Our first victory was won.

That was four years ago. Three years (and counting) past the time her doctor told her she would die.

When you hear the rest of her story, you will cry tears of your own— and maybe, for the first time you will feel hope for yourself or your loved one. But first, let me introduce you to the program that saved Linda's life.

The COPD Solution is a comprehensive, 10-step program for managing life with chronic lung disease. It bridges the gap between merely surviving, or just "getting through" each day, and completely thriving. It's about treating, educating, and implementing lifesaving modifications for anyone suffering with COPD.

THE COPD SOLUTION—A PROGRAM THAT REALLY WORKS

I developed the COPD Solution in a pulmonary rehabilitation facility a few years ago for two reasons. First, there is a general lack of information available for patients, to help the progression of their health and to reduce the deterioration of their condition. Second, I needed a program that could be tailored individually to my patients—their specific needs, routines, abilities, desired outcome, family, and lifestyle.

I'm happy to say that, having used this program with hundreds of patients, the results have been amazingly successful! Impressive to physicians, patients, and their families was how completely life-changing the program was for everyone involved. What surprised everyone was that there is a *100 percent success rate* with those who followed the program.

While it is not a cure for COPD, everyone benefited from its focus on its simple methods to obtain optimal well-being. Patients were able to recapture their lives, and family members gained their loved ones back.

Not unlike assembling a puzzle, with each day and week that passed, these patients put another piece of their lives back together. In the medical world, certain results are expected when one puts certain actions into play. Generally speaking, if you are going to perform a particular procedure on a patient, or recommend a particular type of care, science dictates what the physical outcomes will be. I knew what I expected to take place physically with these patients. I knew what to do to help "fix" their body. However, emotions are different. They have far too many variables to truly be able to anticipate results. When working with individuals, all of whom are so different—they come from different backgrounds, have different life experiences, and cope with things in different ways—it stands to reason the emotional impact of any action can vary widely. So, I was not prepared for the overwhelmingly positive changes that took place. The emotional and mental improvements patients experienced during participation in my program moved them upward in leaps and bounds. Someone who once saw no reason to get up in the morning and had lost all hope in life was now laughing and enjoying friends and family again. How do you place a value on that?

The program itself guides you through every aspect of living with your COPD condition and addresses virtually all situations that may arise. Making your way through this maze may be new, or not. But there are a few things that are universally consistent with everyone I have treated and spoken with, worldwide, regardless of how long ago or recent their diagnosis was made. They are:

1. A need for greater education. There is, universally, a drastic lack of education about COPD and lung illnesses, and such a small percentage of patients have any sort of solid base of knowledge of what they are suffering from, let alone how to successfully live with it, properly and safely administer medications, use of oxygen, specific safety measures, return

to enjoyable sex, and so much more, or that it is possible to do so. With this book, you will become much more informed about your condition.

2. Overwhelming and debilitating anxiety and depression: *when you can't breathe, nothing else matters.* These patients experience this firsthand, every day. When going to the bathroom becomes life-threatening because your oxygen levels drop too low upon doing so, your perspective changes real quick. When it becomes so difficult to eat a meal that you avoid eating on a regular basis, things change. When you can't shower, clean your house, go to work, walk to your car, do your shopping, and more, life reaches an entirely new level of difficulty, and anxiety and depression can become overwhelming. Oftentimes, they are the prevailing feeling of your minutes, hours, days, weeks, and eventually years. Hopelessness, the most dangerous feeling of all, sets in.

3. Disengagement from life and activities. This creates a very real sense of loss, promotes lack of physical activity, encourages deconditioning (loss of muscle tone), and worsens the already present depression.

4. A continual decrease of physical condition, resulting in loss of function.

All these factors inevitably contribute to what I refer to as the COPD Downward Spiral—deterioration of physical, mental, and emotional well-being, all feeding one another in an extremely negative way. You probably know this battle well: It is a spiral that everyone with COPD or a chronic lung condition must battle to escape, even when doing so is necessary to sustain life.

The Bad News

- COPD is the third leading cause of death worldwide.
- It reached that position eight years sooner than projected.

Combined with the number of people also affected by asthma, as well as the over two hundred or more restrictive lung diseases on record, these figures are frightening and overwhelming.

The Good News

- COPD, although considered to be a chronic, debilitating disease, *can* be controlled and *can* be managed, and its progression *can* be slowed down.
- So, if you (or a loved one) have been diagnosed with COPD, your general well-being and prognosis *can* improve *greatly* with proper treatment, education, and care.

My program is the best nonpharmaceutical, comprehensive program available for COPD patients to utilize in conjunction with the treatments their physician has already prescribed and offers profound results, especially when done correctly and completely. It's simple: This treatment saves lives. And this book is a complete pulmonary rehab program you can use in the comfort of your own home at your convenience.

Let's get back to my patient, Linda—who had given up on life and was preparing to die, the same Linda that could only walk 330 feet with multiple rests and dangerous oxygen levels. This program—the proper tools—enabled her to successfully complete the following exercise routine regularly:

- Ride a stationary bike at level 12 resistance for 45 minutes
- Walk on a 5% incline at a speed of 2.5 to 3.0 miles per hour for 30 minutes
- Perform weight-lifting exercises
- Perform standing exercises with ankle resistance weights
- Perform balancing exercises and successfully and safely balance on one leg—even with her eyes shut
- Perform upper body exercises with resistance training
- Perform stair climbing training
- Participate in a regular yoga program
- Control her oxygen levels and keep herself safe

She also made the following changes:

- Lost 30 pounds of fat and gained back 10 pounds of muscle—a phenomenal achievement for her blood oxygen consumption!
- Learned the correct way to breathe and how to properly manage her coughing and mucus
- Successfully altered her diet to include healthier foods, providing proper nutrition for her condition—and learned what foods to avoid!
- Modified her home to allow for optimal oxygen use
- Managed her low blood oxygen moments without having panic attacks
- Shifted from her hopeless emotional state to one of excitement and happiness
- Shared her story with other COPD patients to give them hope

Linda became a person who smiled constantly, cooked her own meals (and meals for her family, especially Sunday and Thanksgiving dinners!). She was able to do her own grocery shopping and laundry, and clean her own house. But even better: she was able to take up her gem-hunting hobby again—an activity that takes all day in the sun, surrounded by dirt—an amazing conquest for her. She also made thirty patchwork quilts in one year for charity as well as three for weddings, two for babies, and one for each member of her family. And she drove to see her son twice last year, with a whole car full of toys for her baby granddaughter. She also drove her handicapped, blind mother on a four-week vacation to see family 800 miles away that she hasn't seen in over ten years.

We shared many, many more triumphs—too many to mention here. And the exciting thing is that her story is not unique.

I could tell you about Jim, the farmer who had almost given up on raising horses (and was as hopeless as Linda when he started), and how he came in one day smiling ear to ear, ecstatic as he announced that he had just washed his tractor all by himself—something he hasn't been able to do for years.

I could tell you about Jan, who is on 6 liters of oxygen per minute to keep her oxygen levels at norm during rest, and how she went from

Write It Down!

While the information offered in this book is not intended to replace the advice of your physician, it can be used in conjunction with and as a supplement to that advice. Sections will provide you with a "Write It Down!" prompt, a tracking system for the many things you will need to organize, from doctors' phone numbers to test results to medications you are taking. You can record these things directly into the forms provided in the Appendix (pages 285–307) or by photocopying the forms to write on (tip: store them together in a distinctively colored folder or binder in a dedicated location, such as where you usually sit to read your mail), or keep your own journal of notes based on the topic suggestions in the Appendix. Getting into the habit of gathering all the important details in one place will make it easier for you to personally review your progress as well as to provide family and your health-care providers with accurate, up-to-date information at the flip of a page.

You can also refer to our website (www.thecopdsolution.com) for additional information regarding your care and to hear questions from other people who are just like you.

trembling with fear to laughing and joking for what is now her hour-long walk.

I could tell you about Sarah, who sang in church for the first time in years and how she cried about it, or how she was so happy to be strong enough to make tortillas for her family again that she brought me some. Or Sarah's husband, who, through tears, thanked me as he told me she was starting to eat again.

Or about Betty's daughter, who flew in from three states away to thank me for bringing her mom back to life.

There are so many stories I could share. But now, it's time to focus on your story. My hope is that you or your loved one will also have a success story after following this program. Ready to get started?

CHAPTER TWO

What Is Lung Disease?

Always remember . . . your focus determines your reality.

—GEORGE LUCAS

Chances are that when you experienced your first real breathing difficulties, it piqued your curiosity as to how your lungs work. We tend to question a bodily process only when things don't work the way they should. But whether you have wondered about it once or a hundred times, it is important for you to understand the physical design of your lungs and the way they operate. This way, you will be able to wrap your head around the disease process your lungs may be in right now, and why they may not be working as well as they once did.

Having an understanding of your body's incredible design will help you more clearly visualize what your medications and therapy are actually doing. You'll understand how air is moving in and out of your lungs, why you breathe the way you do, what regulates your breathing, and what the deficiencies are, so you can do what can be done to improve function. Knowing all this will help you stick to the program, and the more you learn, the more it will help you to make important decisions regarding your health. Remember, the choices you make can lead you toward improvement—or a worsening condition.

HOW DO YOUR LUNGS WORK? THE ANATOMY OF YOUR CHEST

Your chest cavity houses your lungs. It is bordered by your rib cage all the way around, and your diaphragm across the bottom.

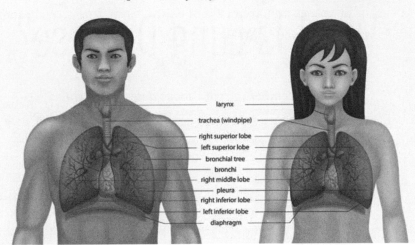

Human Respiratory System (Male & Female)

larynx
trachea (windpipe)
right superior lobe
left superior lobe
bronchial tree
bronchi
right middle lobe
pleura
right inferior lobe
left inferior lobe
diaphragm

Your **diaphragm** is the major "breathing" muscle. When you inhale, it lowers, which changes the pressure and space in your lungs, pulling air into the space. When you exhale, the diaphragm lifts, and the air is forced out of your lungs.

The **pleural space** is an enclosed space between your lungs and your chest wall. It is protected to ensure your lung space is maintained accurately. It doesn't allow extra air inside, thus maintaining the right amount of pressure so that your lungs will expand correctly when you breathe.

Your ribs are wrapped with muscles called the **accessory muscles**. Accessory muscles help lift and expand your rib cage, allowing for assistance in breathing.

You have two **lungs**. Each lung is broken down into **lobes**. The right lung consists of three lobes, and the left lung consists of two lobes. The left side is slightly smaller because your heart is angled to the left of your chest cavity.

Your lungs are full of **airways** and **air sacs**. The airways begin at your trachea (in your neck) and branch out just like a tree into smaller and smaller "branches," all the way through your lungs. At the end of each airway are air sacs called **alveoli** (al-vee-oh-lie). The alveoli look similar to a cluster of grapes and are made of elastic tissue that stretches and retracts with each breath you take.

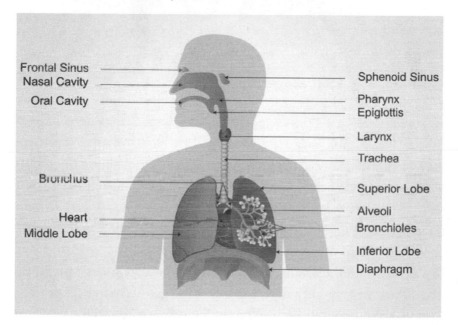

What happens when you have lung disease? When you breathe, you rely more on the accessory muscles to lift the rib cage up and out upon inhalation, and down and in upon exhalation. These muscles are recruited because, as lung disease progresses, it is common for the diaphragm to remain distended as air is trapped in the lungs, leading to a chronic state of hyperinflation. This then limits the amount of movement the diaphragm has, which makes it harder for the air sacs to fill with fresh, oxygenated air.

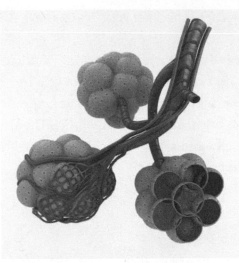

In normal, healthy lungs, the air sacs are elastic and enlarge when you breathe, allowing the surface area on each sac to increase with each breath. The flexible sacs are surrounded by blood vessels. When you breathe in, the sac stretches and expands the way a balloon does when you blow it up. When you exhale, the sac shrinks and retracts back to its normal, deflated size. When those air sacs expand, oxygen is transferred through the tissue into tiny blood vessels called capillaries that surround the air sacs, while carbon dioxide is transferred from your blood back into the alveoli for exhalation. The capillaries around the alveoli resemble a web, and this is where the **gas exchange** takes place. This way, there is a continuous flow of fresh oxygen for your tissues and a continuous release of carbon dioxide from your blood. You might be interested to know that if all of the alveoli were to be removed from the average human's lungs, laid flat, and stitched together like a quilt, the result would be approximately the same size as a tennis court!

With all those air sacs, how can it be so hard for you to breathe?

THE EFFECTS OF LUNG DISEASE

Generally speaking, there are two categories of lung disease—**restrictive lung disease** and **obstructive lung disease.** (COPD falls into the second category.) Within each, there are several diseases that can alter your lungs' function. Lung disease has consequences that go beyond the boundaries of your lungs. You may or may not suffer from some of these issues, which can include:

- Peripheral (arms and legs) muscle dysfunction
- Respiratory muscle dysfunction
- Cardiac (heart) impairment
- Skeletal (bone) disease
- Sensory deficits
- Psychosocial dysfunction
- Nutritional deficiencies

These complications can lead to such things as loss of muscle tone, malnutrition, effects of hypoxemia (not enough oxygen), respiratory muscle fatigue, and frequent hospitalizations. There can be side effects from various medications. Finally, you might also experience psychosocial dysfunction, resulting from anxiety, depression, guilt, dependency, or sleep disturbances. Let's review the two different classes of lung disease—restrictive and obstructive—to gain a better understanding of what may be happening inside your chest.

RESTRICTIVE LUNG DISEASE

Restrictive lung disease "restricts" the ability to breathe similar to the way a girdle inhibits your ability to expand your lungs. An example of this would be scoliosis, or a curvature of the spine. The lung is physically restricted, resulting in a lessening of lung function.

There are many more restrictive lung diseases than there are obstructive. In fact, the list of restrictive lung diseases is very lengthy. For our purposes, we will focus on only a few of the most common ones. We will review diseases that cause an alteration in the lung tissue due to inflammation or scarring. These are called interstitial lung diseases (ILD). These diseases make it difficult for gas exchange to take place from the alveoli to the capillaries because they affect this area of tissue between the two.

Occupation-related ILDs include the following:

Asbestos exposure	Silicosis
Berylliosis	Coal worker's pneumoconiosis
Hardmetal fibrosis	Talc pneumoconiosis

Connective tissue ILDs include the following:

Rheumatoid arthritis	Scleroderma
Systemic lupus erythematosus	Mixed connective tissue disease
Sjogren's syndrome	
Ankylosing spondylitis	Behcet's syndrome

Unclassified ILDs include the following:

Pulmonary fibrosis	Nonspecific interstitial pneumonia
Bronchiolitis	
Bronchiolitis obliterans	Interstitial pneumonitis
Lymphocytic interstitial pneumonitis	Sarcoidosis
	Eosinophilic granuloma
Pulmonary tuberculosis (TB)	Acute pneumonia
Neurofibromatosis	Amyloidosis

ILDs are a diverse group of illnesses with varied causes, treatments, and prognoses. If you have been diagnosed with one of these diseases, your pulmonary rehabilitation educator will offer you information specifically designed to meet your needs and will work with your physician to determine what course of action is most well suited for your care. Common treatments for these diseases include corticosteroids, oxygen therapy, avoiding further exposure, vaccinations, and pulmonary rehabilitation (PR). PR is important in building aerobic fitness, maintaining physical activity, and preventing the musculoskeletal side effects of corticosteroids. In some cases, lung resection or transplantation is necessary.

Diseases that involve respiratory muscle dysfunction are also classified under restrictive lung disease. Such conditions as muscular dystrophies, congenital and metabolic myopathies, anterior horn cell disease, and neuromuscular junction disease are all examples of diseases that involve respiratory muscle dysfunction. By decreasing the ability of the lung to function, ventilation is decreased, and, although their lung tissue itself may be undamaged, patients have a decreased ability to breathe. Treatments for this disease vary depending upon the circumstance, severity, and individuality of each case.

Obesity can also contribute to restrictive lung disease. Fat, especially around the belly, can decrease the diaphragm's ability to function. Over 50 percent of adults in the United States are considered overweight or obese. As the primary breathing muscle, proper function of the diaphragm is vital to a healthy body. Several secondary diseases may accompany obesity. People who are obese are less likely to lead an active lifestyle, are more inclined to suffer from such diseases as sleep apnea, and tend to have poor nutritional habits and engage in reduced aerobic activity. The less you can tolerate activity, the less the lower lobes of the lungs are used. An inactive lifestyle oftentimes leaves the person with a weakened immune system. These factors can lead to greater possibility of lung infections, such as pneumonia, which can further damage the lungs. Sleep apnea can lead to extreme daytime sleepiness and high blood pressure, among other effects, but in many cases can be reduced, or sometimes eliminated, by weight loss.

As you can see, restrictive lung disease can affect us in many ways, inhibiting the function of the lung and the ability for the sufferer to breathe correctly. Whereas restrictive lung disease is hampering the ability for us to breathe from what is often the outside in, obstructive lung disease interferes with the ability to breathe from the inside out.

OBSTRUCTIVE LUNG DISEASE

The other type of lung disease is obstructive lung disease. Obstructive lung disease "blocks" air from flowing in and out of the lungs in a normal, healthy way. Imagine you are driving down a road. Now imagine a boulder falls onto it; it's much more difficult to travel on that road. This is what happens to your lungs when something gets in the way of the airflow. Many things can obstruct airflow, such as mucus in the airway, dysfunctional tissue, or inflammation or reduction in cilia (little hairlike structures that help move foreign objects and mucus through your airways). When your airway diameter is reduced by half its normal size, you would think it would decrease your ability to breathe by half, making it twice as difficult to move air through it. But actually, it

COPD

Why is chronic obstructive pulmonary disease (also known as chronic obstructive lung disease, or COLD) absent from the list of obstructive lung diseases on page 26? This is because COPD is not a disease unto itself; rather, it indicates that several obstructive diseases are acting in tandem. Any combination of two or all three of these specific diseases will lead to a diagnosis of COPD:

Asthma   Emphysema
Chronic bronchitis

Because more than one disease is involved, your symptoms may be heightened or more complex than if you were to have only one of these three diseases.

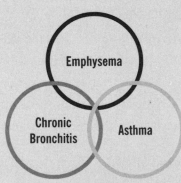

If you have COPD, you may have one of several symptoms:
- Shortness of breath
- Chronic cough (either productive or dry)
- Excess mucus production

becomes *sixteen times* more difficult to breathe when your airway is half as big around! Now you can see why any obstruction in your airway has a large impact upon your ability to move air.

There are only a few obstructive lung diseases. They include the following (COPD, not listed here, is any combination of at least two of the first three diseases; see sidebar on page 24):

- Tightness in your chest, or a feeling that something is stuck in your chest
- Wheezing (high-pitched, whistlelike sound) when you breathe
- You may feel the cold weather more than you used to
- Pollution may affect you more than it used to
- You may notice a change in the way you breathe now compared to how you used to

With COPD, there may be other "comorbidities," meaning you might already have or be more prone to other illnesses, some of which may be chronic.

Have you ever felt overwhelmed by all the different symptoms of COPD? If so, you are not alone. Living with COPD means learning to adjust your life to your new abilities, learning to control your disease, taking your medications regularly, and as directed, pacing yourself, conserving your energy, and practicing daily the things you learn in this book.

COPD is managed with the use of long- and/or short-acting bronchodilators, inhaled or oral steroids, and, if necessary, allergy control to help if asthma is one of your components. See pages 127–168 for more details on medications.

Remaining active may be difficult, but remember that it is vital to your health. Activity, combined with the recommendations your doctor makes and becoming familiar with your body and symptoms, will provide you with the best possible scenario for coping with your disease process. It is a change, but you can do it!

Asthma   Cystic fibrosis
Chronic bronchitis   Pneumonia (although not a
Emphysema   chronic disease)
Bronchiectasis

All of these diseases inhibit the flow of oxygen through the airways by obstructing them with inflammation, secretions, dysfunctional tissue, or a combination of these factors. Let's touch on each disease so you understand what is happening beneath your ribs. Although there are many more restrictive lung diseases than there are obstructive, the medical community tends to place greater focus upon obstructive lung disease because of its prevalence and the level of debilitation and difficulty that accompanies it.

Asthma

The first disease that can be part of COPD is asthma, a disease that affects the airways. If you suffer from asthma, your airways become tighter or are inflamed and swollen. They also make excess mucus. The walls of the airways have muscle in them, and in asthma, those muscles can go into spasm and close down on the airways. Any of these changes make it more difficult to breathe, to get air in and out of your lungs.

Asthma is treated with bronchodilators (rescue breathers) and inhaled corticosteroids, as well as allergy medication, if appropriate. If you suffer from asthma, it is important to be familiar with your medications and what they are used for (see "Asthma 'Steps,'" page 27). This will ensure your asthma is being treated effectively and properly.

The best way to avoid asthma flare-ups, also known as exacerbations, is to steer clear of your triggers and take your medications as prescribed. Treat your asthma as you would a sunburn: The same way you apply sunscreen for a day in the sun, take your controller medications regularly; the same way you would monitor your skin for redness, monitor your symptoms each day by using your peak flow meter and following your asthma education plan; and just like you would go inside when the sun gets to be too much, use your rescue breather when indicated.

That all sounds easy to do, but, to truly understand it, let's take a closer look and get more familiar with what is involved.

Asthma "Steps"

Asthma severity is broken down into steps. Your physician will help you establish what step you are on, and what medications you may need, by reviewing and analyzing your symptoms. For more on these medications, see page 132. And for an explanation of FEV1, the FEV1/FVC ratio, and other tests of pulmonary function, see pages 44–48. For more on exacerbations, see page 154.

Intermittent Asthma (Step One)

- Symptoms are occasional (sometimes seasonal) and experienced less than two times per week. Because they are not regular, you do not need medication all the time or all year long to control them.
- Activities are not limited due to your asthma.
- Your FEV1 is greater than 80%, and your FEV1/FVC ratio is normal.
- Medications will be a short-acting bronchodilator containing Albuterol, and you have to use it less than two days per week.
- Your nighttime awakenings are fewer than two nights per month due to asthma symptoms.
- Your exacerbation risk is one time per year.

Mild Persistent (Step Two)

- Symptoms are somewhat regular, but not daily and not more than three times per week.
- Activities may be limited in a minor way.
- Your FEV1 is 80% percent and your FEV1/FVC ratio is normal.
- Medications include a short-acting bronchodilator, which is used three days per week, and a lowdose inhaled corticosteroid.
- You are awakened three nights per month due to asthma symptoms.

- Your exacerbation risk is two times per year.

Moderate Persistent (Steps Three and Four)

- Symptoms are regular, and you experience your symptoms daily.
- You experience moderate limitations in your activities.
- Your FEV1 is 60% to 80% and your FEV1/FVC ratio is reduced by 5%.
- You use your rescue breather every day and are prescribed a medium-dose inhaled corticosteroid or a low-dose inhaled corticosteroid and a long-acting bronchodilator. You may also be prescribed a medium-dose inhaled corticosteroid and a long-acting bronchodilator.
- You may also be taking other medications, such as theophylline or zileuton.
- Your nighttime awakenings are two nights per week or more, but not every night.
- Your risk of exacerbation is three times per year.

Severe Persistent (Steps Five and Six)

- You experience symptoms all day long, every day.
- You suffer from extreme limitation in your activities.
- Your FEV1 is less than 60% and your FEV1/FVC ratio is reduced by more than 5% of normal.
- Your rescue breather is used several times per day, and you also take a high-dose inhaled corticosteroid and a long-acting bronchodilator. You may also be taking oral steroids to help control inflammation and omalizumab if your asthma is aggravated by allergies.
- You also suffer from nighttime awakenings all week long.
- Your risk of exacerbation is more than three times per year.

Part of controlling your asthma symptoms is to track your symptoms, your triggers, and your medications. Taking the prescribed medications as recommended will ensure optimal opportunity to follow through with this tracking. Starting on page 290 you will find charts to assist you in tracking these important values.

Asthma Triggers

Triggers are those things that cause your asthma symptoms to rear their head. Reaction to a trigger usually initially happens within thirty minutes of exposure and then again at about eight hours after exposure. Keep these time frames in mind when you are reviewing the possible triggers you have been exposed to.

Collectively, some primary triggers in the air seem to be most common: allergens and irritants.

ALLERGENS

An **allergy** is created as a result of exposure to a biological element that your body does not want inside it.

Allergens are biological substances that elicit a chemical response in your body, triggering the release of certain chemicals and causing a response. It has the potential to cause a variety of reactions, from a rash to breathing difficulties, to rhinitis (stuffy, runny nose), to edema, and more.

Each living element in existence has protein markers on its outermost shell that identify it like a name badge. Sometimes your body recognizes these elements as foreign, unacceptable visitors. When this happens, your body essentially launches an attack against the unwanted visitor. This attack recruits defenses that ultimately result in your allergic response to whatever the foreign body may be. That's when you experience an increase of symptoms.

A few major allergens are the most commonly reported as major contributors to increased symptoms in asthma:

Mold (pink, white, black, or green): Mold spores travel through the air and into your respiratory system. They are hardy and withstand most efforts to kill them. Spores protect themselves better than other forms of life.

Cockroaches: If you live in an urban area, this could be a big problem. Watch for evidence of these invading your home, especially if you live in an apartment or condominium where the housing is together or extremely close. The chance of their presence is greater in these types of living spaces. Try to keep the kitchen clean and crumbs swept up, lids on tight, and your garbage and sinks as clean as possible. Watch for droppings. If you find them, call an exterminator as soon as possible. Remember to tell him about your asthma in case his method of extermination requires you to be out of the house for a few days.

Rodents: Mouse urine is another prevalent problem in urban areas. If you notice droppings or find other evidence of mice, such as holes in the walls, cupboards, or floorboards or sounds in your walls, call for help to remove them.

Dust mites: Dust mites are actual microscopic bugs that live in your bedding and mattresses. They eat flakes of dead skin, and their droppings can be especially irritating to an asthmatic. The best way to control your exposure to dust mites is to use a mattress cover with a plastic backing, encase your pillows in proper plastic cases underneath your regular pillow cases, and wash your sheets and blankets regularly in either hot water or cold water with bleach. It is good to dust the area around your bed with a wet cloth (so you don't throw droppings and dust in the air around you). Vacuum at least once a week with a vacuum cleaner that comes equipped with a HEPA filter. If you happen to have stuffed animals on or around your bedding, wrap them in plastic and place them in the freezer for six consecutive hours per week. This will kill the dust mites that may have made your furry stuffed animals their home.

Seasonal allergens: For many, pollens and ragweed are strong proponents of asthma. If you find your asthma gets worse seasonally, and suspect an allergy to pollen but haven't been tested, it is a great idea to speak to your physician about allergy testing. During this testing, small areas of your skin are exposed to allergens to check for a reaction. Once your allergens are determined, therapy can begin to reduce your reaction through a series of shots that expose your body to small amounts of these allergens. With time, you will most likely see improvements in your symptoms upon exposure to these particular allergens. Until then, you can find out what pollens are in the air by watching your local weather channel (or looking online). Most of them have a pollen count during the high pollen seasons, which can alert you to the level of pollen in the air and give you some indication as to what your exposure will be. If you know that, you can decide if you should stay indoors during parts of the day and enjoy the outdoors when the pollens aren't flying so much.

IRRITANTS

An **irritant** is something that you are exposed to in the air that causes discomfort. It does not elicit an allergic response because it is not a biological substance. Look at it like this: If you run sandpaper against your skin, your skin will be irritated, but it is not an allergic reaction. If you rub poison ivy or oak on your skin, your skin will probably be allergic, not irritated.

Cigarette smoke, smoke from a fire, chemicals, wood particles, dirt, paint fumes, and so forth can irritate your asthma. You may have a different reaction to these things than someone else may have. These can all be triggers; the irritation can cause a swelling in your airways, bronchospasm (a spasm of the airways that causes coughing), and other symptoms of your asthma.

The interesting thing is that regardless of what *causes* the symptoms to increase, the result is the same. Asthma is a disease that is always present. The only difference is the

Write It Down! My Asthma Triggers

Your doctor can help you determine what your triggers are, but you can support that by writing down what took place right before your flare-up occurred. Referring to notes you take can help you determine what may be triggering your asthma, and thus help you stay away from things that are bothersome. Keep track of your asthma triggers in the chart on page 299 in the Appendix, or in a journal.

degree to which the symptoms are active. That is why it is important to keep track of and know what your triggers are.

Chronic Bronchitis

The next disease that can contribute to COPD is chronic bronchitis. Both acute and chronic bronchitis are marked by inflammation in the bronchial tubes (the lining of your airways), excess mucus production, and cough. Chronic bronchitis occurs when bronchial tubes become inflamed through irritation. When this happens, function decreases and the production of mucus increases. Inflammation and excess mucus lead to hoarseness and coughing, and make it harder to breathe. Just like asthma, there are outside elements that lead to chronic bronchitis. Smoking, pollution, and environmental allergens can all contribute.

Acute bronchitis is usually the result of an infection in the respiratory tract, caused by a cold virus, flu virus, or bacteria. Chronic bronchitis is most often caused by **cigarettes** or by **inhaling dust or chemicals**. Whereas acute bronchitis caused by an infection can be treated with antibiotics, chronic bronchitis is not treatable with antibiotics. Bronchitis is not an infection; rather, it is a process caused by irritation. While that irritation may be due to infection, it can also be caused by the irritants mentioned above. The best way to prevent and avoid chronic bronchitis is to avoid the irritant causing the bronchitis, drink plenty of water to thin the mucus and keep it from itching, try to control the cough, and take any medication (probably bronchodilators, steroids for inflammation, expectorant and possibly medications to thin your mucus) your doctor has prescribed in the correct manner.

If you have chronic bronchitis, you may also experience a greater amount of mucus production. This can lead to coughing as well that will make you more prone to infection. Your body will have to work harder to exhale. Breathing exercises, such as those on page 103, will help with this. The combination of these processes can lead to shortness of breath, and you may find it more difficult to perform daily activities. Pacing yourself is important. Avoiding irritants can help slow the progression of this disease. If you presently smoke, speak to someone about tools you can use to help you quit. Take medications (long-short-acting bronchodilators or steroids) as directed, and stay active. Exercise can help your body consume oxygen in the most efficient manner possible.

Symptoms of emphysema include:
- Chronic coughing with phlegm production
- Shortness of breath
- Wheezing and recurring colds or illness
- Decreased exercise tolerance

Emphysema

The last disease that can be part of COPD is emphysema. Emphysema is usually caused by inhaling toxic gases, but there is one form of emphysema that is genetic and can affect children called alpha 1 antitrypsin deficiency (more on that later). In both cases, emphysema causes destruction of the air sacs (alveoli). As stated earlier, alveoli are made up of elastic tissue that stretches like a balloon when you breathe. With emphysema, the walls between many of the air sacs are damaged, causing them to react more floppily (like a stretched-out balloon). This destruction of the sac walls also leads to fewer and larger air sacs instead of many smaller ones. When this takes place, two things happen:

1. The air sacs' surface area is lost, which decreases the ability for gases to exchange. As a result, your blood gets less oxygen and carbon dioxide cannot be exhaled.
2. Air trapping occurs. With emphysema, it takes more effort to exhale. This can cause the smaller airways, which are opened by pressure changes, to collapse sooner than they used to. Without the ability to retract like it used to, the tissue cannot help the air get out of the lung. This "air trapping" results in stale air remaining in the alveoli, leaving less space for healthy, oxygenated air to enter. Because of this, over time

your lungs and even your heart may become enlarged. This sometimes leads to what is called a "barrel chest."

Alpha 1 Antitrypsin Deficiency

While cigarette smoking is the major cause of emphysema, a second well-acknowledged cause of emphysema is a genetic protein disorder called alpha 1 antitrypsin (A1A) deficiency. Alpha 1 antitrypsin is a protein that actually inhibits another protein called neutrophil elastase. When the lungs are inflamed or infected, neutrophils, a type of white blood cell, rush to help, and neutrophil elastase is expelled.

If a sufficient amount of alpha 1 antitrypsin is present, the neutrophil elastase is counteracted, which prevents the digestion of lung elastin. Lung elastin serves to protect the lung tissue. When alpha 1 antitrypsin is scarce, the lung elastin is not guarded, and the neutrophil elastase goes unchecked. This causes a failure of the elastin and results in destruction of the alveolar walls, creating emphysema. If this genetic emphysema is present, onset is oftentimes early, even affecting children in some cases.

A1A deficiency is believed to be a drastically underrecognized condition. Only approximately 100,000 people in the United States have been diagnosed; however, it is estimated through current studies that up to 50 percent of current COPD patients are actually living with this disorder but have not been tested. The testing for this genetic component can be important for you and for your family to know. If you have been diagnosed with COPD and emphysema, your physician should do a simple serum test to check for it. If the result is positive, your immediate family members should be checked, as well, as you may share the genetic trait.

In addition to the symptoms of traditional emphysema, there are some symptoms unique to A1A emphysema:

- Yellowing of skin and eyes, or jaundice
- Swelling of abdomen or legs

- Vomiting of blood (from enlarged vessels in esophagus and/or stomach)
- Year-round allergies
- Nonresponsive asthma
- Elevated liver enzymes
- Bronchiectasis

Other Obstructive Lung Conditions

The following disorders are not COPD but are other types of obstructive lung diseases that can damage breathing ability.

Bronchiectasis

Bronchiectasis is a condition that damages the airways, causing them to widen and become flabby and scarred. It usually occurs as a result of a serious lung infection early in childhood, injuring the walls of the airways or preventing them from clearing mucus.

Our airways are lined with tiny hairs called cilia. These cilia help to move particles and mucus from your airways. In bronchiectasis, these cilia are damaged, leading the mucus that builds up to become even more stuck and difficult to remove. Because the mucus remains in the airway, and is warm and moist, it becomes a breeding ground for infection. This often leads to repeated, serious lung infections. Each infection can, in turn, cause more and more damage to your airways. Over time, the airways can lose their ability to move air in and out, which can prevent oxygen exchange from taking place.

Bronchiectasis can affect just one section of one lung, or it can affect both lungs. There are usually no other symptoms except persistent, productive coughing. Postural drainage can help you remove and expel the accumulated mucus. With bronchiectasis, it is important to stay on top of lung infections. Let your physician know if you experience fevers or changed symptoms as soon as you can to treat any new infections and prevent further damage from occurring.

Pulmonary Hypertension

Some people with advanced COPD have a condition known as pulmonary hypertension. *Hypertension* is a fancy word for "high blood pressure." *Pulmonary* is a fancy word for "lungs." So, pulmonary hypertension is high blood pressure in the arteries of the lungs. This is neither an obstructive nor a restrictive lung disease, but it is a diagnosis that can be treated with some of the same treatments as those diseases, such as pulmonary rehab. You may ask yourself, How does this affect me and what does it mean? Let's review the anatomy of the human heart to illustrate the implications and complications of pulmonary hypertension.

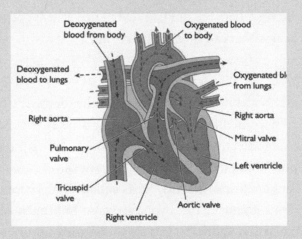

Our heart has four chambers, or rooms, within it, which are called atriums and ventricles.

Arteries and veins lead blood toward and away from your heart, respectively. Looking directly at the heart, you will find the vena cava, the largest major vein that carries blood back to your heart and enters in the upper right side (right atrium) of the heart. This blood is deoxygenated and is coming back to the heart to be pumped back through the lungs to receive oxygen and start the cycle all over again.

The route of blood flow is into the right atrium, through the tricuspid valve, and into the right ventricle. From here it travels through the pulmonary valve into the lungs, where it is oxygenated through traveling around your air sacs (alveoli). Returning to the heart into the left atrium, it travels through the mitral valve into the left ventricle. Now oxygenated and ready to return to your tissues, it exits the heart via the aortic valve, into the aorta (primary or largest artery), and branches off into arteries to be carried to your tissues. After gas exchange takes place at the cellular level in your tissues, your blood is returned, through vessels, back to the vena cava to begin the process over again.

The problem occurs when the blood goes through the pulmonary valve and enters the pulmonary artery on its way to the lungs. In pulmonary hypertension, these pulmonary arteries have increased blood pressure. This means that for some reason the blood running through the arteries meets resistance, and pressure builds. It's now more difficult for the blood to travel through those arteries because they don't expand to allow the heart to pump the blood through very easily. In fact, it can be very taxing on the heart to do this, so you understand how the right side of the heart in a person with pulmonary hypertension becomes overworked.

If the right side of the heart is continually pumping blood through arteries with high blood pressure and is constantly meeting resistance, this causes the heart to work harder. Since your heart is made of muscle, and if you work a muscle hard, over and over again, it will become larger; the right side of the heart consequently enlarges. At this point, heart failure, or cor pulmonale, involves the right side of the heart.

These symptoms and signs may indicate the presence of pulmonary hypertension:

- Ankle and leg swelling
- Dizziness or fainting
- Fatigue or weakness
- Increased abdomen size
- Chest pain or pressure
- Cyanosis (bluish coloration of lips or nails)
- Abnormal pulse
- Larger than normal neck
- Feeling heartbeat right over breast bone
- Liver and spleen swelling

All may be in the presence of normal breath sounds.

Pulmonary hypertension is a chronic disease. There is no known cure right now. The goal of treatment is to treat the primary disease, if there is one, to control those related symptoms. Then efforts will be focused on controlling direct symptoms of pulmonary hypertension with the use of appropriate medications, if needed. For those who suffer from low blood oxygen levels, oxygen therapy is recommended. Your doctor will decide which treatments apply best to your particular situation.

If you have pulmonary hypertension, there are a few additional precautions for you to take:

- Avoid pregnancy.
- Avoid high altitudes.
- Stop smoking.
- Avoid heavy exertion.

Your prognosis will depend upon your specific case and set of circumstances. Talk to your doctor, nurse, and therapist about any questions or concerns you have.

Cystic Fibrosis

Cystic fibrosis (CF) is a genetic disorder affecting the whole body that causes mucus to be thick and sticky. Most people who are born with CF are diagnosed within the first two years of life. A rare condition, it is estimated that only approximately seventy thousand people worldwide suffer from CF. In the lungs, the thick, sticky mucus can block the airways and build up in the airways. This can make it more difficult to breathe and cause persistent coughing and wheezing (that high-pitched sound upon exhalation, like a whistle). When these blockages occur, the lungs can get infected easily, which can lead to damaged alveoli, bronchioles, and bronchi (airways).

If you have CF, it is important to keep the lungs as clear as possible. Using antibiotics, doing breathing exercises, using postural drainage techniques, and drinking plenty of fluids are important. Your medications will probably include aerosol therapy and bronchodilators. Exercise is a fantastic way to keep your lungs healthier. It exercises your breathing muscles and helps move the sticky mucus so you can cough it up.

Pneumonia

Pneumonia occurs when there is fluid accumulating in the air sacs of your lungs. There are different types of pneumonia, or to put it better, different routes in which to acquire it.

Community-acquired pneumonia (CAP) occurs outside hospitals and other health-care settings. CAP is usually acquired by breathing in germs that live in the mouth, nose, or throat.

Hospital-acquired pneumonia (HAP) occurs during a hospital stay for another injury or illness. This generally occurs in patients who use a ventilator during their hospital stay. It is caused by exposure to bacteria or fluid via the ventilator circuit.

Aspiration pneumonia occurs when you accidentally inhale food, drink, vomit, or saliva from your mouth into your lungs. This can sometimes cause pus to form in a cavity of the lung. This cavity is called a lung abscess.

Atypical pneumonia can be caused by several different types of bacteria and is usually spread person to person.

Fungal pneumonia is caused by inhaling the spores of certain fungi. Most people exposed to these fungi don't get sick, but some do require treatment.

Other names for pneumonia include pneumonitis, bronchopneumonia, nosocomial pneumonia, walking pneumonia, and double pneumonia. Most cases of pneumonia are mild, and most people generally get better after one to three weeks without treatment. After you have pneumonia, you may suffer from shortness of breath and fatigue, and some people require the assistance of oxygen for some time. This can sometimes be permanent but usually is not.

Understanding where your lung disease originated and what is happening because of it is an important step to understanding the way you feel and how to best handle your disease and its effect upon you, your life, and your family. As you will learn in the next section, and may discover to be true about yourself if you stop to think about it, many of the symptoms of chronic lung disease happen slowly, over time. You may be able to reflect upon a time not so long ago when you could climb that set of stairs without thinking twice about it,

Write It Down!
My Health-Care Providers

Many people have several different medical specialists overseeing various conditions. Keeping track of who they are and their contact information and specialty is sometimes confusing. The chart on page 285 in the Appendix will help you organize this information into one easy-to-use location for you to refer to. It would be a good idea to carry a copy of this in your purse or wallet in case of an emergency.

whereas now it seems much more difficult. Understanding why you have felt the way you have felt and struggled with some of the things you have struggled with can help alleviate some of the anxiety and emotions you may have been experiencing. Let's talk more about diagnosis and where to go from there.

CHAPTER THREE

Getting Diagnosed

You have power over your mind—not outside
events. Realize this, and you will find strength.

—MARCUS AURELIUS

Lung tissue loses function slowly. Lung disease is not one of those things you just wake up to one morning. Because of its slow onset, lung disease can sometimes go unnoticed until the disease becomes more severe and the symptoms interfere with your daily life enough to prompt you to visit your physician. The symptoms of lung disease can also be confusing. They can point in the direction of other diagnoses and can sometimes be overlooked or unrecognized. Your doctor will be able to tell you whether your symptoms are due to lung disease or something else.

Over time, you may notice a decrease in your ability to perform tasks. Basic activities, such as walking, showering, dressing, or eating, may become more difficult to perform. You may experience a feeling that you just aren't able to get enough air when you breathe. The deterioration of the lung function usually begins years prior to the symptoms' appearing. Have you begun to alter your lifestyle to fit your symptoms? Has your overall immunity been affected by your illness? Are other factors affecting your ability to breathe? Ask yourself the following questions:

Sarah's Story

My very first patient in rehab was named Sarah. She was a sweet lady whose favorite things could be found within three things—serving her family, going to church, and singing while she was there. She was very sick and had begun to make plans for her passing. In addition to her physical illness she suffered from high anxiety and depression had set in. She had been told she would die within a few months' time and she thought participating in therapy was a waste of what time she had left. Sarah's children and grandchildren were her greatest source of pride and she spoke of them often. One of her "hallmark" things to do for them was to make them tortillas. This is something that she had been unable to do for some time now, it was just too taxing on her, left her too breathless, and made her too tired. After a few visits of working with Sarah, I could see her begin to improve. First, it was her activity level, then her attitude, then all of a sudden she began to become more conversational. She was pulling out of her downward spiral and continuing on her upward climb. As more time passed, the changes seemed to come more quickly and more pronounced. One day Sarah came in for her appointment and her grin was spread from ear to ear. "I SANG!" she almost yelled to everyone in the gym. "I went to church for the whole time and I sang all the songs!"

This, to her, was a miracle. Soon to follow was another miracle . . . she made tortillas for her family. This made her even more excited and the shift from the person she was when we began to the woman who came smiling in my office that day was nothing short of a miracle. Her husband, who came to every appointment with her, helped her to the car after her therapy that day and then came back in to talk to me. There were tears in his eyes as he took my hand in his and thanked me for giving him his wife back. I reminded him that I only gave her the tools she needed and that the real work was done on her end. He just repeated his thanks again: She is eating again, she is singing, she is making tortillas. She is alive again! Then he wiped his cheek as he walked back to his car to take his wife home.

- Do I regularly take the elevator instead of the stairs due to shortness of breath?
- Do I have to take breaks and do things in stages due to shortness of breath?
- Is my shortness of breath worsening?
- How long does it take me to recover when I feel short of breath?
- Does my chest feel tight?
- Do I cough up more mucus now than I have in previous months or years? If so, when did this mucus production begin?
- Do my muscles feel weaker?
- Do I limit my time out of the house more than I used to, due to coughing or a lessened ability to exert myself?
- Do I contract colds or flu more frequently than I used to?
- Have I been losing weight?
- Am I subjected to risk factors (tobacco, occupational dust/chemicals, other smoke, etc.) that affect my breathing?

DIAGNOSING COPD

Speaking of diagnosis, there are tests to be done. (Don't worry, they don't hurt!) Once you visit your physician with your list of symptoms, he or she will most likely order diagnostic testing and evaluations to assess your lung function. These may include anything from pulmonary function testing, chest X-rays, and an arterial blood gas evaluation to your medical history, a physical examination, and a survey of your risk factors. These will be used together to help determine the function of your lungs. Here's a rundown:

Pulmonary function test (PFT): This a noninvasive diagnostic test that measures airflow and lung function. It is done by breathing into a special machine while it records its measurements and performs calculations of your results. Greater detail to this testing will be discussed in the next section.

Chest X-rays: Chest X-rays are done to get an inside look at your lungs. X-rays will help identify what may be causing your difficulty in breathing.

Arterial blood gas (ABG): The ABG is an invasive yet simple test done by drawing blood from your artery and evaluating the components in the sample drawn. In obtaining an ABG, your health-care provider can measure with greater accuracy the levels of gases in your blood, which, in reference to lung disease, helps in diagnosis and treatment.

Medical history: You can provide medical history in combination with your medical records to establish symptoms and lifestyle that may help your medical provider understand more clearly what is happening inside your body.

Physical examination: Your health-care provider will conduct a basic physical examination to look for signs that can help lead to a diagnosis.

Evaluation of risk factors: Risk factors play an important role in your lung disease. Risk factors such as smoking history, environmental history, symptom history and severity, and indoor and outdoor pollution must be reviewed.

PULMONARY FUNCTION TESTING

A pulmonary function test measures how well your lungs work. There are three areas of study in a PFT. These tests measure:

Symptoms That Require Urgent Care

Please contact your physician or go to an emergency room immediately if you experience any of the following symptoms or situations.
- Rapid heart rate
- Inability to "catch your breath" while talking
- Loss of mental alertness
- Discoloration of lips
- Discoloration of nail beds
- The recommended treatment for your symptoms isn't working.
- Your symptoms worsen.

1. How much air your lungs can hold in **volume** and **capacity**
2. How quickly the air moves in and out of your lungs
3. How efficiently the gas exchange (oxygen into your blood from your lungs and carbon dioxide from your blood into your lungs) takes place

> ### Write It Down!
> ### My Symptom Tracking Chart
> See page 290 of the Appendix for a chart into which you can record any of the aforementioned symptoms you have personally experienced, so you can report them to your physician.

The combined results from all three areas provide a calculable picture of your lung function. Remember that PFTs, on their own, cannot diagnose a specific disease. They provide your physician with results that can help determine what *type* of disease you have (restrictive or obstructive) as well as the severity of it. They are also used to determine the effectiveness of medication used to treat lung disease.

Note: Because of the nature of some of the tests, you should be prepared to abstain from taking some of your regular breathing medications for a time prior to the testing. Your physician will give you directions.

Remember, also, that once a lung disease has been diagnosed, your physician will most likely order additional PFTs to follow your progress. The timing for these follow-up tests will be determined by your physician. The knowledge gained from these tests, in combination with the other testing and exams that will be performed, will enable your physician to properly diagnose your symptoms. Results of your

> ### Write It Down!
> ### My New Symptoms
> It is a good idea for you to track symptoms or changes other than just the ones you feel are directly related to your pulmonary care. Track anything you feel is out of the ordinary for you or anything you feel your physician should know about, such as leg swelling, edema, new pain, chest discomfort, and so on, using the chart on page 298 of the Appendix.

PFTs will be good for you to know and understand so you can perform at your optimal function and be at ease with the goings-on.

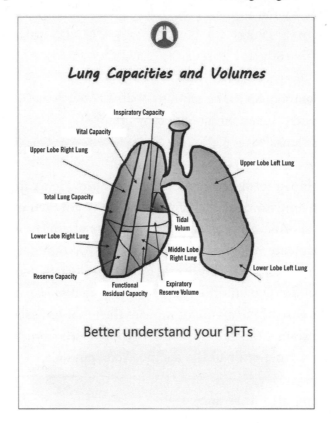

Lung Capacities and Volumes

Inspiratory Capacity

Vital Capacity

Upper Lobe Right Lung

Upper Lobe Left Lung

Total Lung Capacity

Tidal Volum

Lower Lobe Right Lung

Middle Lobe Right Lung

Lower Lobe Left Lung

Reserve Capacity

Functional Residual Capacity

Expiratory Reserve Volume

Better understand your PFTs

What a PFT Measures

When it comes to what the PFT measures, there's no shortage of acronyms. What do they all mean? Here's a cheat sheet.

Your PFT will measure four lung "volumes" and four lung "capacities" and air movement.

Lung Volumes

Expiratory reserve volume (ERV): The difference in the amount of air in your lungs after a normal exhalation (FRC) and the amount after you exhale with force (RV).

Inspiratory reserve volume (IRV): The maximal amount of additional air that can be drawn into the lungs by effort after inspiration.

Tidal volume (Vt): The volume of air you breathe with each regular breath.

Residual volume (RV): The amount of air in your lungs after you exhale completely. It can be measured by inhaling a gas and measuring how much is exhaled.

Lung Capacities

Each capacity measurement is made up of at least two lung volumes.

Total lung capacity (TLC): The total volume of air your lungs are capable of holding after you inhale slowly and deeply. Total lung capacity = expiratory reserve volume + inspiratory reserve volume + tidal volume + residual volume.

Inspiratory capacity (IC): The maximum amount of air you can draw into your lungs. Inspiratory capacity = tidal volume + inspiratory reserve volume.

Vital capacity (VC): The maximum amount of air you can blow out of your lungs after maximum intake. Vital capacity = expiratory reserve volume + tidal volume + inspiratory reserve volume.

Functional residual capacity (FRC): The amount of air in your lungs after a regular exhaled breath. Functional residual capacity = expiratory reserve volume + residual volume.

Pulmonary Flows

Forced vital capacity (FVC): Measurement of the amount of air you exhale with force after you have inhaled as deeply as possible.

Forced expiratory volume (FEV): Measures the amount of air you can exhale with one breath.

> **FEV1:** Amount exhaled in first second of exhalation.
> **FEV2:** Amount exhaled in two seconds of exhalation.
> **FEV3:** Amount exhaled in three seconds of exhalation.

Peak expiratory flow: This measures how forcefully you can exhale. It can be obtained at the same time as your FVC.

Forced expiratory flow 25–75 percent: Measures airflow halfway through the exhalation.

Forced expiratory flow 200–1,200: Measures your exhaled breath between two predetermined points during the FVC.

Maximum voluntary ventilation (MVV): Measurement of the maximum amount of air you can breathe in and out in one minute.

Slow vital capacity (SVC): Measurement of the amount of air you can exhale slowly after you inhale as deeply as possible.

OPTIMIZING YOUR PERFORMANCE OF PULMONARY FUNCTION TESTING

The word *test* can be frightening to anyone. Whether waiting for results or the process of testing itself, the thought of medical tests can be daunting and overwhelming. But it doesn't have to be. These tests don't hurt. Once you understand what it is you are doing, you will be much better prepared to perform each portion of testing. It is important that you stay calm for your test to be performed optimally. Much of what you will do is effort-dependent, meaning that your ability to properly do each test will greatly impact the accuracy of the tests. Anxiety can interfere with your results. Read on for exactly what you need to do to get the most accurate results possible.

Your PFT will be performed in your doctor's office. To begin, you will sit upright and will wear a nose clip to ensure accuracy. To do a spirometry test, which is used to determine the lung volumes, you'll be given a mouthpiece to breathe through. This, along with the nose clip, can be uncomfortable, and it may take you a few minutes to adjust and get used to each device. Your physician should allow a few minutes for you settle in, and encourage you to relax and breathe through the mouthpiece at your normal pace and depth.

Measuring Pulmonary Volumes

Inspiratory reserve volume (IRV): To obtain a measurement of this volume, you will be asked to breathe a few times at regular, quiet volume and then exhale maximally. This will most likely be measured a few times, as well, and the two largest measurements should also be very close, within no more than 5 percent difference.

Tidal volume (Vt): When you are used to breathing through the mouthpiece, you will be asked to continue breathing at a normal, quiet rate for a few minutes. This is the measurement of your tidal volume (regular, quiet breaths). Tidal volumes will change somewhat with each breath. For this reason, an average will be calculated for your tidal volume.

Residual volume (RV): It can be measured by inhaling a gas using nitrogen washout or helium dilution and measuring how much is exhaled.

Expiratory reserve volume (ERV): The difference in the amount of air in your lungs after a normal exhalation (FRC) and the amount after you exhale with force (RV).

Total lung capacity: This is done by adding up all measured and calculated volumes.

Inspiratory capacity: When it is time for your inspiratory capacity to be measured, you will be asked to take a breath at maximum depth after exhaling at a regular tidal volume. You will very likely be asked to perform this several times. The two largest measurements should be very close, within no more than 5 percent difference.

Vital capacity (VC): There are a few methods to measure vital capacity. It can either be measured upon inspiration or during an extended exhalation if air trapping occurs. If you are asked to measure vital capacity upon inspiration, you will be asked to exhale "all the way to empty," or as completely as possible followed by inhaling as deeply as possible. The volume measured at maximal inspiration is the vital capacity. If you are asked to measure vital capacity upon exhalation, you will be asked to inhale maximally and then exhale maximally for as long as it takes you to be "empty."

Functional residual capacity (FRC): This is done by adding the ERV and RV or by performing tests known as nitrogen washout or helium dilution, in which inhaled gases are given and measured through exhalation.

Measuring Pulmonary Flows

Pulmonary flows, or mechanics, are the ability for the lungs to move a volume of air. In measuring this, it is possible to detect obstruction in the airways, both large and small. Measuring pulmonary mechanics includes measuring FEV (forced expiratory volume measured at one, two, and three seconds of an exhaled breath), FEF 25–75 (forced expiratory flow between 25 and 75 percent of exhaled breath), FEF 200–1,200, PEFR (peak expiratory flow rate), and MVV (maximum voluntary ventilation).

FVC: To determine your FEV1, FEV2, and FEV3, as well as your FEF 25–75, you will be asked to inhale maximally followed by an exhalation as quickly and forcefully as possible. This sounds easier to perform than it is. Be sure to ask your provider to demonstrate and explain precisely how they would like you to do it, to prevent yourself from doing it

Nitrogen Washout and Helium Dilution

The nitrogen washout test, although it may sound daunting and scary to some people, is really a rather simple, painless test. It is designed to measure the functional residual capacity of your lungs and airflow. It is designed to help your doctor look for dead space in your lungs. Measuring dead space will tell us how much "stale" air you typically have stored in your lungs. Stale air is air that does not participate in gas exchange, meaning that due to loss of lung function the oxygen in this air and carbon dioxide in the blood don't switch places as they should. If you have a large amount of dead space, it is an indication of poor or decreased lung function and, as stated above, poor gas exchange.

To perform the nitrogen washout test, you will be asked to breathe through a machine that will feed you pure oxygen for a set period of time. Then you will exhale for as long as possible through the same machine, which will read the nitrogen in your air. Normal nitrogen content is 78 percent on room air, so anything above that is measured as the amount of nitrogen you have in your lungs, which represents the amount of dead space you have. It does this because nitrogen is not a gas that is exchanged in the lungs; it is simply a part of the atmospheric air that we breathe, causing it to be a measurable gas when washed out of the lungs with another gas, such as oxygen.

If a healthy set of lungs performs this nitrogen washout test, it would take approximately seven minutes for all the nitrogen to wash out of the lungs. In lung disease, because of loss of lung function, it can take much longer.

Helium dilution is a test that is performed to measure the air in the lungs that participates in gas exchange. It will tell your physician such values as your functional residual capacity, expiratory residual volume, inspiratory capacity, slow vital capacity, and total lung capacity. To perform this test, you will breathe through a device called a spirometer, which will be used to measure the components of the air that you breathe. You will be asked to slowly blow out all of your air until empty, and then return to normal breathing for a few minutes. You will need to blow out all the way to empty and take a slow, deep breath as large as you can tolerate, then to blow out slowly until empty. You will be asked to return to normal breathing for a few minutes before taking out the mouthpiece. Then you can rest.

incorrectly and having to repeat it too many times. You will want to blow out forcefully, without any hesitation, from the very beginning of your exhalation. Do not slow down or stop until you are completely empty.

This test will be performed a few times to ensure accuracy. The largest of at least three tests will be recorded as your FVC. All other quantities, such as the FEV1, FEV2, FEV3, FEF 25–75, FEF 200–1,200, and MVV (discussed as follows), will be attained from the FVC test.

FEV1, FEV2, and FEV3: This measurement illustrates the amount of flow exhaled in each respective time (one, two, and three seconds of the FVC). It is indication of obstruction, and the percentage (gained from a calculation of the FEV/FVC ratio) will help your physician determine the severity of obstructive lung disease.

FEF 200–1200: This test is measurement, in liters per second, of the volume of your exhaled breath between two predetermined points during the FVC.

PEFR: PEFR is a measurement of the fastest point of flow of air during exhalation. Measuring peak flow can be and is sometimes done while measuring FVC but it can also be performed independently of your PFTs by using a peak flow meter. You will find additional information regarding the use of your peak flow meter in the medication section of this book (see page 161). With obstructive lung disease, tracking your peak flows can help you monitor the effectiveness of your medications as well as observe possible exacerbations as they begin.

MVV: Successful measuring of the MVV depends greatly upon how you perform the test. For this test you will be asked to breathe in and out as deeply and as rapidly as possible for 12 to 15 seconds. This test demonstrates the ability of the diaphragm and intercostals (muscles around the ribs) to expand the chest and lungs. It also tests how open or constricted your airways are. The measurements will be recorded, calculated, and converted to a volume in liters per minute.

Slow vital capacity (SVC): This is measured by maximum inhale followed by slow exhalation. This is different from the FVC because the airways will be opened for different lengths of time during each measurement.

What Do Your PFT Results Mean?

After you take your PFT tests, the results will be calculated and returned to your physician, who will follow up with you on what the results mean. When you go for a PFT, be sure to ask how long it usually takes for results to be in, and call your provider's office or schedule a follow-up appointment to go over your results. Don't be afraid to ask questions to clarify and understand what it all means.

You can use the following table to compare your results to what a normal range would be. Patients with COPD typically show decreased measurements in both the FEV/FVC ratio as well as the FEVl. These measurements, in conjunction with your symptoms, will be used to determine the severity of your disease. A management strategy will then be established and treatment will begin.

Normal PFT Results Chart

PULMONARY	NORMAL
Tidal volume	0.5 L
PEFR	8.0 L
Functional residual capacity	3.1 L
Forced vital capacity	5.0 L
FEVI/FVC	80%
FEF 25–75	4.0 L
FEVI	4.0 L
Total lung capacity	5.0 L
Residual volume	1.6 L

Write It Down! My Pulmonary Function Test (PFT) Results

Ask your health-care providers to share your PFT results with you, and turn to the chart on page 286 in the Appendix to record your numbers. As you review your results, be sure to get clarification on what they mean. Never hesitate to ask questions of your providers. They want you to understand the meaning of everything as much as you want to understand it yourself.

THE GOLD STANDARD: COPD STAGES

Now that you have your PFT readings, your physician will have a better sense of how severe your COPD may be. He or she may refer to the Global Initiative for Chronic Obstructive Lung Disease (GOLD) standard as a means to classify the stage of your illness. These five stages are used to guide health-care providers to the therapies and treatments that have been proven effective at each particular point during the disease process.

The GOLD standard of care is a suggestion for therapy, as it stages the level of disease dependent upon PFT readings and associates those levels with particular care recommendations:

0: At risk. Chronic symptoms, exposure to risk factors, and normal volumes. Avoid risk factors.

I: Mild. FEVl/FVC less than 70 percent, FEV greater than 80 percent with or without symptoms. Add short-acting bronchodilators.

II: Moderate. FEVl/FVC less than 70 percent, FEV greater than 50 percent with or without symptoms. Add regular treatment with one or more long-acting bronchodilators and add pulmonary rehab.

III: Severe. FEVl/FVC less than 70 percent, FEVl greater than 30 percent with or without symptoms. Add inhaled glucocorticosteroids if repeated exacerbations.

IV: Very severe. FEVl/FVC less than 70 percent, FEVl/FVC less than 30 percent *or* with chronic renal failure (CRF), and right heart failure. Add long-term oxygen if CRF, and consider surgical treatment.

THE SIX-MINUTE WALK TEST

Your ability to perform your activities of daily life is easily demonstrated to your clinician through how well you can walk—regardless of how far or fast it may be. Of the various walking tests out there, the six-minute walk test (6MWT) is typically better tolerated than other choices, and, because it requires a low level of exertion, it's also more reflective of your ability to perform daily tasks.

The test is done in your doctor or therapist's office. It tests your ability to exert yourself, measuring the distance/how quickly you walk on a flat, hard surface in six minutes. All the space it requires is a 100-foot stretch of hallway. With this simple test, your practitioner will be able to evaluate your pulmonary and cardiovascular system as well as measure your circulation, your neuromuscular system, and your muscle metabolism. (A cardiopulmonary stress test gives more in-depth info on these.) A 6MWT will be done periodically to monitor your progress.

The 6MWT is self-paced, and during the timed test you can rest if you need to. When my patient Linda did her walk test, she had to stop and rest several times—and that's perfectly fine. It's not a race. You are not trying to push yourself to your extreme limits. You are just walking at a pace you determine. During your test you may or may not require the use of supplemental oxygen, depending on what your physician orders.

To perform your six-minute walk test, you will want to do the following things:

- Wear comfortable clothing and appropriate shoes.
- Remove all fingernail polish. (It can interfere with an accurate reading.)
- Use your usual walking aids, such as a walker, crutches, cane, etc., if necessary.

- Eat a light meal prior to morning or afternoon tests.
- Do not exercise within 2 hours of the beginning of the test.

When you are ready, your provider, or the person administrating the test, will have you stand at the starting point. By this time, your vitals (blood pressure, oxygenation, and heart rate) will have been recorded along with your sex, height, weight, age, any medications taken prior to testing, and oxygen (if you are to begin your test with oxygen on).

When you begin your walk, your timer will start and will continue to run through the six minutes while you walk, and even if you rest. Find a comfortable pace for yourself, not too easy and slow, but not too fast, either.

Begin your walk. Make note of where the "turn-around" points are and be sure to follow the course the test administrator has directed you to follow. This will ensure accuracy in calculating your distance.

Continue walking for the entire six minutes, resting on chairs provided for you if you need to. During your rests, the timer will continue. Don't let this panic you; this is how the test is supposed to be. Sit and rest until you are ready to continue. When you feel ready, simply stand up and resume your walk, continuing until either you need to rest again or your time is up. Remember, your heart rate and oxygenation will be recorded throughout your walk. This is routine. It will most likely be taken with an oximeter, which is a little fingertip device that measures the saturation of oxygen on the hemoglobin in your blood. It is noninvasive and painless, but for it to work optimally, all fingernail polish should be removed prior to your testing.

Write It Down!
My 6-Minute Walk Test Results

It is a good idea for you to know and be familiar with your 6MWT results and keep a record for yourself. Comparing records of multiple tests can help you track your progress or perhaps catch a decline in your performance. This can help you be more familiar with your body and your health.

When your walk is completed, your laps—or distance—will be tracked for calculation, and your heart rate and oxygenation will be recorded. You will be asked to rate how you feel based on a scale from 1 to 10. This is the Borg Scale, and next you will find an example of how it works.

MONITORING YOUR EXERTION

The **Borg Scale** is used by clinicians to determine how well you, as a patient, are tolerating activities. It is based solely upon how you feel. Because it is completely subjective, meaning any answer you give will be correct—there are no wrong answers. You can practice using this in all of your activities, rating how you feel for each. This is a great way to track your progress because you will see yourself do more while remaining at the same level of difficulty. Under most circumstances (unless under medical supervision), it is a good idea for you to *not* work yourself to a level 9 or 10. These levels are going to make it very difficult to breathe and should be avoided in your daily activities.

The Borg Scale of Perceived Exertion

0	Rest
1	Very easy
2	Easy
3	Moderate
4	Somewhat difficult
5	Difficult
6	
7	Very difficult
8	
9	Very, very difficult
10	Maximally difficult

IS IT COPD . . . OR SOMETHING ELSE?

Differential diagnosis is a term used when there are multiple possibilities that can be a cause of your illness. With lung disease, there are many possible symptoms each patient may experience, but each case can also be individual. It essentially serves as a process of elimination. Here are some examples of what your physician may be looking for when reviewing your symptoms.

COPD or Other Condition

POSSIBLE DIAGNOSIS	SYMPTOMS
COPD	• Onset in midlife (after 40 years of age) • Symptoms progress slowly • Smoking or environmental exposure • Shortness of breath upon exertion • Airflow obstruction (largely irreversible) • Chest X-ray presents large amounts of air trapping (later stages of disease)
Asthma	• Onset early in life (childhood) • Varying symptoms from day to day • Allergies often present (often accompanied by eczema or rhinitis) • Airflow obstruction (largely reversible) • Possible family history of asthma • Chest X-ray used to rule out other issues
Bronchiectasis	• Onset at any age (usually result of a childhood illness) • Large volume of sputum (likely with a strong, foul smell) • Breathing sounds like coarse crackles (like crisp rice cereal) when physician listens through stethoscope • Usually accompanies a bacterial infection • Chest X-rays present dilated airways
Tuberculosis (TB)	• Onset at any age • Tissue sample confirms diagnosis • Exposure to and prevalence of TB • Chest X-ray presents lung infiltrates or nodular lesions
Congestive heart failure (CHF)	• Breathing sounds like fine basilar crackles when physician listens through stethoscope • PFT demonstrates volume restriction vs. airflow restriction • Chest X-ray demonstrates dilated heart and pulmonary edema (swelling)

CHAPTER FOUR

Introducing the 10-Step Program: What to Expect

Happiness is the meaning and purpose of life, the whole aim and end of human existence.

—ARISTOTLE

Your journey to this place began decades ago while you were busy doing other things. It happened while you were bringing up your children, going to work, and vacationing. It was present during birthdays, anniversaries, and holidays. Many summer nights welcomed it. Some of your journey you actively participated in, such as your education, your career, and your relationships. Other parts took place almost unknown to you, such as the way your heart continued to faithfully beat every day, the way your red blood cells reproduced on their own countless times throughout the last several decades, and the way your brain triggered your breathing without conscious participation on your part. All of these things combined to make you *what* you are right now and to place you *where* you are right now.

If you are reading this book, it is likely that this part of your journey includes a diagnosis of chronic lung disease for either yourself or someone you love. Obviously, you may have many questions and concerns. Your diagnosis most likely came after years, possibly a decade or more, of suffering with the silent symptoms of lung disease. Suffering for this length of time is not uncommon. Because the onset of lung disease is gradual and symptoms increase slowly, most people usually adapt fairly well to the minor changes they notice over a period of several years. Therefore, most people diagnosed with lung disease suffer for a very long time before their symptoms become severe enough to seek medical attention, which is unfortunate, because the best way to treat lung disease is to fight it head on—actively, directly, and purposefully.

This book is designed to help you do just that: evaluate every part of your life regarding your lung disease and grab it by the horns. This book offers you my proven 10-step program. In this book, you will learn:

- Methods to incorporate necessary lifestyle adjustments into your daily life
- Key information on oxygen therapy and other devices
- The importance of pulmonary rehabilitation
- Nutritional education—how food can really affect your health and what to eat to help you feel better
- Why smoking cessation is so crucial—and methods to assist in this difficult, yet vital choice
- Time and energy management
- How to overcome intimacy issues
- And much, much more

In each section you will also find strategically placed tracking resources to help you organize and use everything that is available to you, giving you the ability to streamline your health care, your providers, your medications, and nearly every aspect of your life, to save you time and energy for more important things. This book will also help you learn what questions to ask, and identify what answers to search out. YOU are your best advocate. YOU need to make sure your health-care providers are supplying you with many of the various therapies that will ultimately lead you to the most thorough and precise methods of care designed specifically for you.

Using this much-practiced program and the tools within it will afford you the ability to get your life back and truly live. By learning what you can do to control your symptoms and develop a way of life to grow with your symptoms—all while making minimal adjustments to your lifestyle—you will discover how to keep active and pursue your greatest dreams. This book will guide you toward the skills necessary to effectively manage your disease and your future.

ACCEPTANCE

It is important that you get to a point in which you accept your condition. Remember, acceptance is not resignation but the first step to success. According to Webster's dictionary, to accept something means to receive it willingly; to be able or designed to take or hold; to give admittance or approval to; to endure without protest or reaction; to regard as proper, normal, or inevitable; to recognize as true; to make a favorable response to; and to agree to undertake. Now, compare this to resign: to resign means to give oneself over without resistance, to give up deliberately. So, it is also important that you do not resign yourself to your condition or its symptoms.

Accepting your condition will allow you to progress, make allowable changes to your activities, and alter your previous methods of performing tasks to fit your current situation. If you were diagnosed with diabetes, you would alter your diet to stabilize your glucose levels. If you were diagnosed with hypertension or high cholesterol, you would make the prescribed adjustments to your life to ensure the lowering of your blood pressure or cholesterol. This disease is no different. It is a matter of altering your methods of doing things and finding a "new normal" that fits with your current situation.

Physical symptoms are one thing; the emotional struggles that accompany lung disease are another. Dealing with and gaining a grasp on your emotions is of vital importance to your success. The stages of grief and the role your emotions play in your well-being are part of any journey with a chronic illness. It is important for you to realize that you need to grant yourself permission to feel these emotions and also recognize when your emotions are getting the best of you.

OXYGEN THERAPY AND CPAP/BIPAP MACHINES

At some point in your illness, you will likely be prescribed oxygen therapy—the standard of care for chronic lung disease. You should be careful about using oxygen unless and until you become informed about why it is beneficial to use, how it helps, and what some of the hazards or safety precautions may be. Oxygen comes in a few different forms and uses a few different modes of delivery. You will learn about it all, from safety to storage to personal care. Your anxiety will flee, and you will become more comfortable and at ease with your oxygen use. Oxygen is, after all, the essence of life.

You also may have heard of or been asked to use a CPAP or BiPAP machine. You will find this book stresses the importance of using these items, as well. As with anything else you use, a thorough understanding of what type of conditions CPAP and BiPAP are recommended for, how their use could benefit you, and what changes you can expect to see if you use them will be included. Managing anxiety is also an important part of this therapy and can be achieved through trial and error of different masks and products. Your comfort is also essential.

BREATHING TECHNIQUES

As I've said before, "When you can't breathe, nothing much else matters." This book is full of breathing exercises that will help you relax, rejuvenate, and revive. You will also learn how to expel your excess mucus most appropriately and effectively.

LEARNING TO RELAX

There are so many things you can learn to do to conserve energy and make the most of your efforts. You can improve the efficacy of what you already do, and find ways around the things that seem so difficult. These changes are now of vital importance to you. Every day. The most important thing you can do is pace yourself.

You will learn that relaxation is now one of your highest priorities, and why. You will also find multiple positive self-statements to help you prepare for both emotionally charged situations (which immediately affect your breathing) and times when you feel short of breath, offering you reassurance that you will make it through. Building up your "emotional self" is essential to both your present and future trials. It will help you deal with anxiety, prevent panic, and gain confidence that you are capable of handling these difficult situations. You will see some yoga poses that help you breathe better and improve overall well-being and learn how and why the practice of this art is beneficial to you.

MEDICATIONS, MEDICATIONS, MEDICATIONS

There can be so many medications, and keeping track of them all can be so challenging, especially when they are all scheduled at different times during the day, need to be taken in the correct order, and need to be used in the correct method to receive the most benefit. You will gain a complete understanding of what, when, why, where, and how for each of your medications. You will also learn to track different aspects of your medication regimen to keep your health-care providers informed and yourself educated on what your "normal" is and whether your medications are helping you maintain a state insufficient to meet your demands. This will also help by providing you with a visible warning that a decline may be on the horizon.

PULMONARY REHABILITATION

Pulmonary rehabilitation (PR) is a program designed to assess and treat the emotional, physical, occupational, social, and nutritional issues that arise as your body deals with the effects of your lung disease. It is a program based upon addressing your physical need as to activity through weight and endurance training, as well as specific physical therapy exercises that may address your own special needs such as balance, joint, pain relief, and other ailments that affect your ability to perform the regular activities you need to do on a daily basis. It will also focus on breathing retraining, so you can learn how to effectively breathe with your lung disease, and yes, it is different than you are used to doing. A good PR program will offer community support and an opportunity to spend time with others who are familiar with how you feel. This generally leads to building friendships and relationship building that is healthy for you, as you can share concerns and difficulties and talk about ways to work around those things. As recent changes in health care have reduced both your access to this care and coverage for it, this book can be used as a guide to your own special PR program and help you learn how to incorporate these things into your daily life.

QUITTING SMOKING

One of the first things your rehab team will cover is smoking cessation. If you are still smoking, quitting cannot be stressed enough. I'll cover a few different methods to try, medications that will help, replacement therapy, withdrawals, relapse, triggers, reasons to quit, and a "quitting contract" that helps psychologically with quitting and encourages your success. Quitting is the single best thing you can immediately do for your health.

NUTRITION AND LIFESTYLE

Another immediate thing you can do for your health is remember that food is medicine.

You will discover foods that actually make your breathing more difficult—as well as those that will help you feel better, learn the COPD Cycle of Malnutrition, and find tracking sheets that will enable you to better organize your efforts in the kitchen. Using pacing and energy-saving methods to cook and plan will take you far.

STAYING CONNECTED

When you're suffering from a chronic disease, intimacy with your spouse or partner can be difficult or complicated. There are ways around the difficulties you may need to adjust to. Rest assured it is not only possible to maintain an intimate relationship with your loved one, but it can still be rewarding, as well. I offer some tips and suggestions for helping you and your partner to adjust to your new normal.

Step by step, you *can* overcome your COPD. Here are just a few comments from patients who have successfully completed the COPD Solution program and their loved ones:

> *When I started this program I didn't think I would ever do anything again, I had decided I was going to die. Now I am gem hunting again, walking around the block, quilting, and traveling. It works! It saved my life!*
>
> —LINDA, PARTICIPANT

> *These lessons are so useful. Full of information I could not live without!*
>
> —JUDITH, PARTICIPANT

> *When I started, I couldn't do anything. I had to sell my chickens because I couldn't walk far enough to feed them. Now I am walking every day, lifting weights, and riding my new road bike outside. It even has a basket for my oxygen tank.*
>
> —ROBERT, PARTICIPANT

> *The information is so interesting to know. Every time I go through it I learn something new.*
>
> —ROY, PARTICIPANT

The lessons learned, and the time Dawn spent with my mother are priceless. Her program has changed our whole lives. I don't know what my mother would have done without it, but I know she wouldn't be with us today.

—FAMILY MEMBER OF A PARTICIPANT

PART II

THE COPD SOLUTION PROGRAM

Make Peace with COPD

It's the gymnasium of life where you get the work-out, the resistance, and you find things out about yourself that you didn't know.

—BISHOP T. D. JAKES

So, you have lung disease. You may have just received your diagnosis, or you may have been diagnosed years ago. Either way, you are most likely struggling with such symptoms as shortness of breath when you exert yourself; trouble breathing; feeling like you're not getting enough air; a chronic, persistent cough with mucus or a dry cough that won't go away; possible pain upon exhalation; and fatigue. Prior to a COPD diagnosis, people may endure these symptoms for years, commonly leading to increased severity of the disease, worse symptoms, and delayed proper medical attention.

Lung disease is often stressful. If you've been diagnosed with COPD, then you need to know that the emotions you are experiencing as well as the changes you are facing are normal—you *are not alone*. Millions of people around the world feel the same way you do each morning. They have a chronic cough that often produces mucus, which can be embarrassing. They have a medication regimen similar to yours and understand the time it takes and the routine you must establish. They can relate to how it feels to require the use of oxygen every day. They know how hard it can be to do things that used to be so simple and miss having the ability to perform those activities. They share your frustration in making the lifestyle adjustments their symptoms have required of them.

Living with chronic lung disease means you have already made, or will at some time be required to make, some difficult lifestyle adjustments. This *does not* mean that life cannot be enjoyable, and it *does not* mean you will have to stop doing all the things you love to do. What it *does* mean is that you may have to modify the way you do them.

One thing my patients have found to be very helpful is to write down their thoughts, feelings, concerns, and questions. You may also want to keep a dedicated journal or use your computer; whatever is easiest for you. While sometimes it's not easy to share feelings with your family, friends, or your doctor, getting them out on paper can help. Give yourself ample time to think about how you are feeling. This will be your first lesson in pacing yourself. This isn't a race; there is no rush to the finish line. Patience, pacing, and persistence are your new best friends. As you review the subsequent steps in this book, you will learn to understand that *life is now all about these three things*. Writing these notes to yourself will be your start.

Since your diagnosis, or perhaps even prior to your diagnosis, you may have been struggling with how the changes in your body have affected your life. Such changes inevitably bring upon each of us varying degrees of emotion, which may include some or all of the following feelings: fear and anxiety, depression, confusion and frustration, anger, disbelief, grief, and concern for the future.

Let's review some of these emotions, some causes, and some solutions for each. The change a chronic disease diagnosis such as this may carry with it is the need to process what might feel like an insurmountable pile of information and emotions. Such change usually, to some degree, causes us to grieve. Grieving is a normal process that should not be ignored but instead understood.

> ### *You Are Not Alone: Finding Support Groups*
>
> Please understand that you are not alone in feeling these emotions. There are reasons for them, and, while they are not all the same for everyone, they are all common. It is important for you to reach out and discover that others around you feel the same way. The American Lung Association sponsors Better Breathers clubs; you can find one in your area by going to www.lung.org/lung-disease/copd/connect-with-others/better-breathers clubs/ (or just go to www.lung.org and search for Better Breathers). Your health-care provider may also be able to recommend support groups in your area to help you cope and boost your spirits. There is great power in realizing you are not alone, in having someone to share your burden and ease your struggle.

FEAR AND ANXIETY

Lung disease attacks the very most important thing you do: *breathe.* Difficulty breathing complicates your ability to function in every way, and with good reason. Your lungs are the delivery system for oxygen to get to get to your blood—the pathway to your cells. Oxygen is the very essence of life. Not being able to breathe has to be one of the scariest things there is. For this reason, anxiety is extremely common for those suffering from lung disease.

Located deep within your brain is a center whose sole responsibility is to monitor your breathing. It is constantly monitoring the levels of different gases in your blood, regulating your breathing rate and depth. It is constantly looking for something to be "wrong," triggering your body to fix what it perceives to be broken. One of the functions your brain uses to encourage your body to fix problems it senses is to create a feeling of anxiety within you.

When you feel anxious about school or work, you are driven to do what is necessary to succeed. When you feel anxious about getting your finances in order, it nudges you to work toward that goal. This anxiety has good intentions, prodding you to alter what you are doing, encouraging you to repair what is out of balance, which will send your brain a message of relief. But when anxiety is constant, its effect can be the opposite—paralyzing.

In the case of lung disease, and the corresponding breathing difficulties, a feeling of suffocation or claustrophobia is most often the root of your anxiety. It can be triggered by odors, smoke, elements in the environment, an activity, and—believe it or not—emotions themselves. Ironically, your anxiety makes your feeling of suffocation worse. We will discuss in later sections what to do to "reset" that feeling of suffocation and ease your anxiety.

The first thing to do is to realize that:

1. You are not alone: this response is normal.
2. You are not crazy: the difficulty is real.
3. And, finally, there are things you can do to help yourself feel better.

Anxiety Can Be Paralyzing

You've heard the expression *fight or flight*. This is biology's way of helping you cope and find a healthy balance in managing your anxiety levels. When you enter the fight-or-flight mode, certain things happen within your body. These things work to your advantage in an emergency, but in the long term it can be detrimental to your health.

Your mind and body are connected—what you think and feel directly affects your health. When your brain notices a stressor, your body physically reacts. In the short-term stress response, your body secretes endorphins (chemicals in the brain). The physiological responses to these endorphins are increased blood glucose levels for energy, blood vessel constriction that forces your blood to take oxygen to your vital organs, increased metabolic rate, numbing of pain, and dilation of the airways. This reaction is designed to help you remove yourself from an emergency situation. As soon as the emergency is over, your body is signaled to relax and your blood vessels and breathing patterns return to normal. In situations where you need to do something in the short term to protect yourself, this stress reaction is good. It happens, and then it resolves. But when stress becomes an ongoing issue, the anxiety itself becomes a problem for your health, especially when you have another condition, such as chronic lung disease.

With long-term anxiety, the body secretes extra hormones on an extended basis. The kidneys retain fluid, blood volume and blood pressure increases, proteins and fats are broken down for energy, there is an increase in blood sugar, and the immune system gets suppressed. This can lead to a variety of health problems. Unrelieved stress can have a drastic effect on your wellness and ability to function. For those with COPD, anxiety is especially difficult because it often dramatically affects breathing patterns. When breathing is difficult it compounds anxiety, which, in turn, causes more difficulty breathing! Managing your anxiety is therefore essential to your well-being. Don't let your anxiety paralyze you. Practice how to handle the short-term anxiety so it doesn't become a chronic problem for you or your health.

THE STAGES OF GRIEF

With a diagnosis of COPD, you are dealing with a great change, one that may significantly alter many things in your life. You will have to make changes in the way you do things. If you haven't yet, you will have to start listening to your body's needs. Pacing and planning are now essential in your daily and weekly activities. All of this information—these piles of letters and words and notes and directions—can feel overwhelming. As you adjust to all of this, one of the first things you must realize and give yourself permission to do is grieve.

We often hear of people enduring the six stages of grief, as identified by Elisabeth Kübler-Ross. This seems to most commonly be referred to in conjunction with the death of a loved one, but the same stages also apply to most major changes and significant losses in our lives. Now, considering the changes that you may experience with this diagnosis, these stages may apply to you as you adjust to your diagnosis and its symptoms. At some point in time, you will most likely experience all of them, as will your friends and family members. Although the original model is five stages, I've adapted it to reflect the stages that my patients go through.

Although most people's basic emotions during the grieving process are the same, everyone processes each stage and emotion a little differently. Realize that your family members, in many cases, will be experiencing and processing the same emotions, but you may experience each stage at different times. Also, remember that progressing through these stages is not a neat and smooth adventure. It is messy. It can feel unorganized. It may involve traveling back through previous stages or ahead to others, as it may not be done in direct order. Please consider these things as you review these stages:

- Denial, shock, and disbelief
- Guilt and frustration
- Anger and bargaining
- Depression and loneliness
- Reflection, reconstruction, and working through
- Acceptance and hope

Denial, shock, and disbelief: Even if you haven't felt well for some time, you may react to your COPD diagnosis with some element of shock. You may be unfamiliar with the terminology you hear and what the disease means. You may not believe the reality at some level, so as to avoid the pain. Shock serves to provide emotional protection to us from being overwhelmed all at once. This may last for weeks.

Guilt and frustration: As the shock wears off, it can be replaced with the pain of guilt. Although sometimes excruciating and almost unbearable, it is important that you experience the pain fully, and not hide it, avoid it, or try to escape from it. You may have feelings of guilt or remorse over lifestyle habits or other things you may or may not have done to bring this on. Life can sometimes feel chaotic and scary during this phase.

Do you have that added stressor of guilt on your plate? It's like eating that extra piece of pie after a holiday meal—your mouth waters as the pie looks up at you from the plate, all warm and covered in delicious homemade whipped cream. Scooping bite after bite into your mouth and savoring the taste and texture, your brain releases endorphins that flood your bloodstream and make you feel good—until it's over.

That is when the pants feel too tight, the discomfort sets in, and the calorie counting starts, along with the guilt. Does it do you any good to dwell on the guilt that piece of pie brought you? Not really. Does it do you any good to focus your energy on the pants that feel too tight, knowing you may have very well brought this on yourself? Not so much. What is done is done. Undo your pants, make the adjustments you need to be comfortable, and let it go. Because you can't remake those decisions, frustrating as it is. You can only make better decisions in the future.

If you acquired this lung condition from years of smoking, *let it go*. If you have lung disease from years of working in conditions of dirty air, *let it go*. If you are stuck to an oxygen tank because you lived with a smoker for years, *let it go*. There are mounds upon mounds of reasons for why you could have lung disease, including genetic reasons—which you could do nothing about. Living with guilt is like dragging around an anchor—and it has been proven that this extra "weight" can have a direct negative effect upon your physical condition. Do not burden yourself with guilt. *Let it go.* Doing so will enable you to focus on the present and the steps you need to do now to take care of yourself.

Taking care of yourself in the present, without the burden of guilt, will enable you to relieve some of the frustration you may also be experiencing. With guilt removed from your mind and heart, you'll be free to focus on performing new exercises specifically designed to help these emotions. In so doing, your concern for the future will also be brought into check, and you will experience the capacity to not only enjoy life right now but realize that you have life left to enjoy. Many patients feel as if this diagnosis (and the list of medications that seem to be a mile long) is equal to a death sentence. With work and training, many of those same patients grow to understand that life is still here, looking you in the face every single day. It is attainable. It is enjoyable. And it is a very liberating moment when you discover for yourself that you can still "live."

Anger and bargaining: Frustration eventually gives way to anger. You may lash out and lay unwarranted blame for your diagnosis upon yourself or someone else. You may question fate, asking, "Why me?" Or you may try to bargain with the powers that be for a way out of your despair. Please try to take control of your emotions by doing such things as journaling your feelings instead of simply stating everything that comes to mind, finding a friend or other safe person to whom you can confide your frustrations, or redirecting into a pleasant hobby or other activity the energy you are wasting in negative emotion. Support groups can be great tools; you'll find other people who know exactly what you're going through. Whichever healthy way you choose to unleash your anger, it will help you avoid permanent damage to your relationships. This is a time for the release of bottled-up emotion.

Depression and loneliness: Just when those around you may think you should be moving beyond the dismay of this diagnosis, a long period of sadness may overtake you. It has been said—and you may have experienced—that depression can accompany major changes in our lives. This is no exception to that rule. You may feel hopeless and that things will never get better.

Even the simplest daily tasks can take much more effort. Lung conditions can make you feel tired a lot of the time. These conditions often interrupt your sleep, and simple things like eating can become exhausting. Some of the medications you take may alter the taste of your food. You may now have to haul oxygen around, which makes some people feel awkward, and you may feel as if your freedom has been limited. If you have a cough, you may feel self-conscious from the noise and mucus production you experience. You may not be capable of controlling your cough the way you would like. You may feel winded and have to rest more often than you would like. You may find shopping trips and excursions need to be planned, and you may miss the spontaneity of just picking up and going somewhere. You may feel some discomfort from your oxygen tubing.

Many of these factors combine to make it difficult for you to want to leave the house and go out much; you may start to feel isolated, as my patient Linda did. If you have spent much of your life being active, this, too, may feel like a huge struggle. All of this puts you at a greater risk for developing depression, so pay close attention to how you feel and how long those feelings last. You need to feel these feelings, so don't let friends and loved ones talk you out of it. While their advice is well-meaning, these feelings are a normal part of the grieving process and you need to be able to work through them. You may realize the true magnitude of your loss. You may be inclined to isolate yourself on purpose in an effort to analyze things. You may sense feelings of emptiness or despair.

Here are some common signs of depression:

- Irritable attitude with everyone and everything in your life
- Difficulty problem solving and concentrating
- Altered appetite, either increased or decreased
- Hopeless feelings—that you will never feel better, no matter what
- Increased crying and crying easier than usual
- Sleeping changes
- Sad feelings for more days than not, for two to three weeks in a row
- Inability to laugh or enjoy yourself
- Low self-esteem, feeling of worthlessness
- Feelings of guilt
- Increased sensitivity to criticism
- Decreased interest in people or activities

If you suffer from depression, you may feel hopeless about your future and disconnected from your life. This happens to many people with a diagnosis of a chronic illness. If you suffer from more than five of the items on the list above, please take time to talk to your physician, nurse, or rehab therapist. Depression can become a very debilitating ailment, affecting both your mind and your body. If you feel there is no hope for improvement, you may struggle to follow any treatment plan. If you feel panicked about your health, you may not use the tools you are being given to improve it. The worse you feel, the less energy you have. The less you want to do, the less you strive to take care of yourself and your condition.

Many patients ask, "After all that I have lost, don't I have a right to feel depressed? Shouldn't I?" The answer is yes, and the answer is no. While it is completely understandable for you to feel a loss right now, it is not natural or healthy for you to remain in that state of despair. There are a variety of treatments available, including medication and psychological counseling. A combination of the therapies may be necessary to offer you optimal relief. Please do not suffer with this alone. Share your burden with those around you who care and want to help you.

Through doing these things, and as you start to adjust to life with your diagnosis, your life will become a little more calm and organized. Your physical symptoms of stress will lessen, and your depression will begin to lift slightly. You will experience the upward turn.

Reflection, reconstruction, and working through: As you learn how to manage your disease and become more functional, your mind starts working again. Tasks that seemed impossible may be a bit easier—you're learning how to do things in a new way. You will find yourself seeking realistic solutions to problems posed by life and the changes that await you. You will start to work on reconstructing yourself and your new life.

Acceptance and hope: During this, the last of the seven stages, you learn to accept and deal with the reality of your situation. Acceptance does not necessarily mean instant happiness. Given the pain and turmoil you have experienced, you may never return to the carefree, untroubled YOU that once existed. Life doesn't usually allow for that. But you will find a way forward. You will find your new normal.

Participating in an effective pulmonary rehabilitation program (see page 169), which will help you cope with your emotional and physical struggles, can be of great benefit to you during this time. A good rehab program will offer you the emotional support you need as you work through these stages, by building camaraderie with fellow patients experiencing the same emotions and physical ailments as you, as well as having access to trained professionals who will be available to answer your questions and concerns.

ALL IN THE FAMILY: DEALING WITH COMMON REACTIONS FROM FAMILY MEMBERS

You may find that your family shares in many of your emotions. You may notice changes in the way your family treats you or reacts to you. Some family members may become overprotective; others may distance themselves. Try to remember that while you are dealing with many changes, so are they, and they may deal with emotions in a different way than you do.

Think about how you feel when someone you love is sick or hurting and you feel powerless to help. For many people, anxiety is a natural response to fear, to the unknown. Your husband or daughter may not know what you are feeling—they may be as scared as you are. Tell your family how you feel and what changes need to be made to accommodate your circumstances. They will appreciate understanding what's going on in your body and the strains those changes have put on you. With that understanding, they will be more familiar with your limitations and will therefore create new expectations for you.

You may be asked such questions or hear comments as:

"You haven't done much, are you tired already?"

"Can't you walk a little farther?"

"Why do you need help with that?"

"It is taking a long time for you to do this."

Try not to get frustrated with family members when they make these types of comments. Instead, take advantage of these opportunities to teach them what it is like to struggle for breath.

There is an exercise you can do with them that may seem silly, but it is guaranteed to help them understand how you feel. Next time you are at the grocery store, purchase a bag of straws. Ask your family member to put a straw in his or her mouth, plug his or her nose, and do something active while breathing through the straw.

While this is different than the *way* you breathe, it is a close comparison to how it feels *when* you breathe. They will become more understanding about your shortness of breath, thus helping them create new expectations for you.

Your family can be a wonderful resource; they can also be a great support. Use them, rely on them, delegate to them when necessary. Together, you can slowly establish what your new normal will be. This may mean varying schedules and activities from what they have previously been, but you will adjust.

HELPING A FAMILY MEMBER WHO HAS COPD

If you have a family member with COPD, you may be asking yourself what you can do to help this person and help your family. Understanding what he or she is going through enables you to better offer physical and emotional support. It will also help you better comprehend your family member's new limits as well as his or her abilities. There are several things you can do to assist the situation.

Be aware of the basic things: Living with the uncertainty that can accompany lung disease can be taxing and difficult. Learn the symptoms you should watch for, signs of respiratory distress or failure (see

Chapter 3, page 43), and medications to use in emergencies (and keep them handy). Become familiar with the health-care team members your loved one has access to. They can be a valuable resource.

Familiarize yourself, if you haven't already, with your family member's health-care services. Become familiar with the facilities that are in network with his or her insurance providers, as well as the pharmacies, physicians, medications, and outpatient services in your area. Ask your loved one to authorize you to discuss his or her health with these people and services, and to be permitted to pick up medications for him or her if need be. This will help alleviate the possibility of extra expenses and save time in appointment scheduling and management. If you need to call the insurance company, or contact someone who may be an expert in this, it would be a good idea to do so.

Read. Listen. Learn. Diving into information from books, the Internet, physicians, and therapists will help you understand the symptoms, physiology, and prognosis of what you are dealing with. Knowledge is power, and can help free you from the sometimes overwhelming anxiety that often accompanies such life changes. Most important, don't forget to call upon family and friends for help. Don't do this all alone.

Take care of yourself, too. It is not uncommon to find it hard to keep perspective on everything that is happening. Caregiving can be a stressful job. If you're feeling overwhelmed or scared, first, allow yourself to feel. Don't ignore these emotions or try to disregard their place. Let them happen. Experience them. Permit them to exist. You deserve it. Second, while you are experiencing these emotions, watch yourself. If you feel you are beginning to dwell in a state of depression or a slump you just can't get out of, ask for help. If you notice yourself experiencing signs of depression (see page 77), especially if you start having trouble eating or sleeping, talk to your own physician or a counselor about how you feel. Ask for the help you need. Caregivers sometimes suffer from periods of isolation. This isolation, aside from zapping your self-esteem, can be a sign that you are overwhelmed.

Find a support group. Just as it is important for your COPD sufferer to feel that he or she is not alone and has the support of others, it is important for you to have an effective support system of your own. There are local and online support groups that are full of people experiencing the same life experiences and emotions you are experiencing. Seek them out. It will help you understand how your loved one feels, understand your own emotions, and learn new methods or ideas to do things that may be very beneficial.

What can you do if you are overwhelmed? Maintaining connections with your church or community group, neighbors, friends, and other family members can often help. Most of your loved ones will be happy and willing to help, once asked. They just need to know you need the help. Take advantage of resources in your community. Try hiring a sitter or an aide, either on a regular basis or just for special occasions; arrange for other family members to take turns providing care. Check into local nursing homes or assisted living centers. Many of them offer respite care for anywhere from a few hours up to a few days. Arrange for other family members or an aide to assist in housework and cleaning. It might even help for you to change your expectations of yourself. For some, that might mean letting the laundry go once in a while or cooking simpler meals. For others, it might mean asking for more help. It is important to realize, also, that for some people, nursing homes or assisted living facilities really are the best option, providing them with professional care that may be beyond your scope.

Last, but not least, incorporate relaxation and meditation into your life. These types of simple activities offer many benefits, which are reviewed later in this book.

Start Oxygen Therapy

Do one thing every day that scares you.

—Eleanor Roosevelt

Many people are surprised to learn that among the prescribed medications they receive to relieve the symptoms of their lung disease is oxygen. Oxygen therapy is a popular and essential treatment for most people suffering from chronic lung disease. It is the most common treatment for respiratory disorders. It has been shown to improve survival and quality of life—and can make a big difference in how you feel.

Clinical guidelines are followed in prescribing oxygen therapy. Let's go back to your pulmonary function testing (PFT), discussed in Chapter 3. If your FEV1 (measurement of flow in your PFT) is less than 70 percent and your FEV1/FVC is less than 30 percent (or if it is in conjunction with chronic renal failure or right heart failure), adding long-term oxygen is the standard of care. Your practitioner will determine your blood oxygen level either by doing an ABG test (see page 44) or by using a noninvasive fingertip oximeter to monitor your hemoglobin saturation (see page 56).

Jan's Story

I have worked with my patient Jan for a number of years. Like most people, Jan's disease crept up on her very quietly over a period of several years. She experienced shortness of breath, coughing, wheezing, and unbeknownst to her, extremely low oxygen levels. She was fatigued, experienced some occasional dizziness, and just wasn't feeling right.

These symptoms led her to visit her primary care physician. Just as at any office visit, they took her vitals first. Her blood pressure was good, her heart rate was high, and her oxygen saturations were . . . 74! That's a far cry from the above-90 standard we try to stay at. The nurse took the oximeter off that finger and tried another. Then she got another machine and tried it on both hands. Every reading was within 2 points of the initial 74. The nurse politely told Jan she would be right back, and did come right back—with the doctor, another nurse, and an oxygen tank in tow. Jan likes to joke that she went into the office feeling like a million bucks and came out on oxygen, wondering what hit her. Her oxygen levels were likely so low for so long that she didn't realize her coloring, energy level, and ability to perform tasks were so altered, and she also didn't realize that her internal organs such as her heart were working overtime to make up for the deficiency.

HYPOXEMIA

To be prescribed oxygen therapy, you must have a condition known as **hypoxemia**—a low blood oxygen level (saturations of less than 89 percent). Most patients with chronic lung disease, at some point, experience this. Some patients do not qualify for oxygen therapy at rest, but may desaturate during sleep or upon exertion, therefore qualifying them for oxygen. For example, I recently worked with a patient who oxygenated well while sitting and even while performing upper body exercises, but as soon as we walked across the room, she would desaturate to the mid-80s or sometimes even lower. Oxygen therapy provides her with the oxygen she needs to perform activities of daily living without putting extra stress on other internal organs. There are no real reasons to not use oxygen therapy as long as the indications are present.

Hypoxemia is the beginning of respiratory failure. Please familiarize yourself with these symptoms so, in case they happen, you will be aware of what may be taking place. It is also a good idea to make your family, friends, and caretakers aware of these symptoms, so they can help you with your oxygen. In fact, you should familiarize them with all of your equipment and ensure they have a complete understanding of how to use your tanks, concentrator, and so forth, in case of emergency.

Hypoxemia Symptoms

SYSTEM	SYMPTOM
Respiratory system	• Shortness of breath • Discoloration (pale or blue/purple around mucous membranes, such as mouth or nose, or discoloration of your fingernails) • Increased heart rate
Cardiovascular (heart) system	• Increased heart rate/rapid heart rate • In severe cases, heart rate may slow down or begin to have arrhythmias (irregular heart rate) • Mild hypertension (increased blood pressure) • Peripheral (arms, hands, legs, feet) vasoconstriction (blood vessels constrict, smaller in diameter) • In severe cases, hypotension (low blood pressure) may eventually occur
Neurological (nervous) system	• Restlessness • Disorientation or confusion/lack of coordination • Headache • Distressed appearance • Blurred or tunnel vision • Slow to react • Impaired decision-making skills/impaired judgment

> ### *Write It Down! My Hypoxemia Symptoms*
>
> If you experience symptoms of hypoxemia, keep track of them in the chart on page 299 of the Appendix. It is important to track these levels because they will help you become familiar with how each level feels, so you will know what your own needs are during different activities and when you desaturate. With enough practice you will be able to guess where your levels are and how much you need to adjust your oxygen liter flow to help you recover. It will also be good to have a record for your physician to know how your current prescription is meeting your demands.

HOW MUCH OXYGEN DO YOU NEED?

Once your physician decides the therapy is necessary for you, he or she will determine what your liter flow will be (in liters per minute, or lpm), or the concentration of oxygen you will require, as well as determine when you need it. After you begin your therapy, you may notice an immediate difference in how you feel. The goals of oxygen therapy are, of course, to correct hypoxemia and the symptoms thereof, and to decrease the extra work hypoxemia imposes upon the body.

You may be prescribed oxygen only at night, during moments of exertion, or as a full-time, 24-hour-per-day treatment. Your condition may be one that requires you to **titrate**, or adjust, your oxygen levels upon activity to keep your saturations greater than 90 percent. *If you do have permission from your physician to titrate your oxygen, it is very important that you remember to turn your liter flow back to your original, resting liter flow when the exertion is over.* Remember that oxygen is a drug, and, as with any drug, there can be negative side effects if not used properly.

As you can see, liter flow determines the percentage of partial oxygen you breathe. Your liter flow is usually determined by your physician. Your liter flow will also help determine which delivery device (cannula, mask, etc.) you will use with your oxygen (more on these later in this

Oxygen Percentage/Liter Flow Chart

ENTRAINED OXYGEN AMOUNT	OXYGEN PERCENTAGE
Room air	21%
1 lpm	24%
2 lpm	28%
3 lpm	32%
4 lpm	36%
5 lpm	40%
6 lpm	44%
7 lpm	48%
8 lpm	52%
9 lpm	56%
10 lpm	>60%

chapter). It is very important that you are familiar with the parameters of your delivery device.

Whether you use a mask or cannula, ask questions of your oxygen company, your therapists, and your doctor. You need to ensure that your liter flow matches your delivery device. For instance, if you wear a simple mask, it is vital that you never have your liter flow set at less than 5 lpm. Wearing a mask increases the amount of oxygen you get from a liter flow by a small percentage, so it can be beneficial for those who have low oximetry levels, but wearing one at a flow rate that is too slow will force you to rebreathe carbon

Write It Down! My Oxygen Use and Activities

If you have permission from your physician to adjust your oxygen levels, depending on your activity, you may need to adjust your liter flow to keep your oxygen saturations above 90 percent, or at the desired, prescribed level. Turn to page 301 of the Appendix and record in the chart what your liter flow requirement is for each activity.

dioxide (CO_2), which contradicts the goal and can be very dangerous. Never hesitate to ask questions!

OXYGEN DELIVERY SYSTEMS

How may you get your oxygen? There are several types of oxygen delivery systems:

- Oxygen concentrators (designed for home use)
- Portable oxygen concentrators (designed for travel outside the home)
- Humidity system (works with a concentrator)
- Compressed oxygen cylinders (tanks of various sizes for walking around or for travel)
- Liquid oxygen systems (can be used in place of a concentrator at home, as well as on the go)

Each system has its advantages and disadvantages. Your physician may have specific ideas of what type of delivery system he or she would like you to use, or you may have the option of choosing which one will work best for your lifestyle and needs. Let's review each system.

Oxygen Concentrators

If you have oxygen at home, you most likely have been provided with a concentrator. A concentrator is a device that plugs into your wall and physically separates the oxygen from the room air (concentrating it) for delivery to you. It has adjustable liter flows, and, through a filter (usually located on the back or the side of the machine), it pulls room air into the machine.

At a liter flow of 1 to 2 liters per minute (lpm), a concentrator provides between 92 and 95 percent oxygen flow. At a setting of 3 to 5 lpm, the oxygen concentration of flow falls to between 85 and 93 percent. Most concentrator output is limited to a 5 lpm flow. Higher flows are usually achieved by running two systems together.

If you require continuous low-flow oxygen, you may find that concentrators are the most cost-effective oxygen supply method. A concentrator in your home will increase your overall energy expenses by only 5 to 10 percent. It is important to remember to clean your filters regularly to optimize the efficiency of your concentrator.

Portable Oxygen Concentrators

The popularity of portable oxygen concentrators (POCs) is growing. They are smaller concentrators mounted on a wheeled frame that can be taken with you when you leave the house. These are increasing in use because of the freedom they offer. There doesn't have to be as much attention paid to the amount of time you will be gone from home because the battery life on the portable concentrators, depending on your liter flow, typically lasts longer than a portable tank. There are also no loading and storing of extra tanks for the trip. Portable concentrators can plug into your car's battery power and remain charged for longer periods of time.

For the most part, these POCs run the same way as the concentrator you use at home, just on a smaller scale. They are ideal for travel and are approved by many airlines. However, although they are very convenient and used by a growing number of the population, they are not for everybody. Be sure to speak with your physician about whether your symptoms will tolerate one. Your oxygen demand is a major decision maker in whether the option may work for you. I have had patients that leave the house with two tanks tied together to have enough liter flow for them to saturate at 88 or greater; in a situation like this, a POC would not be sufficient for demand. Also, depending upon where you are going and the length of time you will be gone, whether you can use the pulse dose setting (conservation setting), or whether you will have access to power to charge the unit, as well as extra batteries for backup, will all be factors in whether this device will be sufficient for you. Not every patient can tolerate the liter flow and method of conservation of POC support. You should also talk to your insurance company to check on coverage for one of these units. Not all insurers will cover the expense of POCs, so you may be left paying out of pocket for one.

Humidity System

Your sinuses and upper respiratory system are designed to warm and humidify the air you breathe before it gets to the delicate tissue of your lungs. When oxygen is forced in through your nose, nature has a hard time doing its job. Your sinuses are very sensitive, and high-flow oxygen can be uncomfortable if you do not have the right supplies. If you are on a liter flow greater than 2 liters per minute, ensure your oxygen supplier has provided you with a humidity system for your concentrator—and instructed you on how to use it. Make sure you keep humidity entrained into your oxygen line. It will alleviate sinus pain (which often feels like a headache), dryness, and nosebleeds from your oxygen.

Whether or not you have a humidity system, rinses and gels can be applied inside your nose and into your sinuses to alleviate dryness. These moisturize the mucus that may be hardened by the increased airflow and/or oxygen. These help with movement of the secretions, clearing your nasal passage of blockages, and protecting the frail layer of skin and tiny capillaries inside your nose. Ask your physician or pharmacist about what products are available for this, and don't be afraid to use them.

Compressed Oxygen Cylinders

Compressed cylinders come in several different sizes and are used for different purposes. Large tanks are used for backup supply or to refill smaller tanks used for ambulation or travel. Some are refillable in the home and some are not. They are usually either placed in wheeled carts or in bags with a shoulder strap or handle to ease carrying.

In the old system, the smallest of these cylinders is the AA tank, and they get progressively larger up to the E tank; a more recent system labels them M plus a number. However, each home care company has its own individual method of labeling tanks, so become familiar with what labels your home care company uses for the tanks that work best for you.

Pressurized cylinders are regulated by pressure-reducing valves with a flow meter, which is needed to regulate the delivery of oxygen. These valves are equipped with adjustable dials that allow for adjustment to your prescribed liter flow.

Liquid Oxygen Systems

Liquid oxygen cylinders can dispense a flow of 0.5 lpm up to 8 lpm. One cubic foot of liquid oxygen is equal to 860 cubic feet of gas and weighs 2.5 pounds. Obviously, liquid oxygen systems can store large quantities of oxygen in a smaller space. At a liter flow of 2 lpm, a small liquid oxygen tank (L tank) can last for up to eight hours. Liquid oxygen is held in a tank with a similar design to a thermos bottle. The inner container of liquid oxygen is suspended in an outer container with a vacuum in between. With the liquid kept at minus 300 degrees, constant vaporization (oxygen gas) always exists above the liquid. When the flow is turned on, the gas passes through a vaporizing coil, where it reaches room air, warming it. It is released and metered through a flow control valve.

DELIVERY METHODS: FROM THE TANK TO YOU

If you use oxygen, regardless of which system you are using, you probably wear a nasal cannula, the most common device used for long-term oxygen delivery to the body. It blows oxygen into your nose by means of a flexible hose ending with two small prongs that sit in your nares (nasal openings). The hose loops around your ears and meets under your chin. Simple masks and conserving (reservoir) masks are sometimes used, but not as commonly as they must be used with a higher liter flow than the cannula demands.

Studies have shown that most of the oxygen is taken in during the first half of each breath. If this is true, the oxygen administered by continuous flow during the last half of each breath and exhalation is wasted. Using a conservation device, which can conserve the oxygen in the tank by 30 to 50 percent, can offer you more freedom and time with your travel tanks, making your therapy both more efficient and less intrusive—true therapeutic benefits! There are a few different types of conserving devices:

Demand flow devices: Demand flow (also called pulse dose) devices operate by using a flow sensor and valve to synchronize oxygen delivery with your breathing rate. It dispenses a burst of oxygen whenever it senses the pressure change at the beginning of each breath. If your physician feels you can tolerate the use of a pulse dose meter, he or she will most likely adjust your liter flow to approximately half of what the continuous flow is prescribed at, and adjust it according to your tolerance, monitoring your saturations through oximetry (most commonly used) or blood gas analysis.

Reservoir devices: A reservoir device is used to trap oxygen from a continuous flow system that would otherwise be lost. The oxygen accumulates during expiration, allowing you to use this otherwise wasted oxygen. This reduces the amount of oxygen released to you and more effectively uses what is readily available.

Reservoir devices can reduce the loss of low flow oxygen by 50 to 75 percent; for example, using such a device, a patient who is on a liter flow of 2 lpm could feasibly oxygenate on 0.5 lpm, which extends the tank life significantly.

Although the flow saving is predictable, there are factors that may affect it, such as nasal anatomy and breathing patterns. If you use any of these reservoirs, remember it is essential for you to exhale through your nose. This reopens and resets the reservoir membrane. Exhalation through pursed lips may impair performance, as well, especially during exercise. For these reasons, it is essential to thoroughly evaluate your tolerance level for these devices.

TAKING CARE OF YOUR EQUIPMENT

It is important to remember to maintain your tubing, cannula, or mask. Watch for discoloration and stiffness or a brittle feeling to your tubing. Replace it when the discoloration or brittleness occurs. Also, reservoir cannulas will need to be replaced approximately every three weeks. (This somewhat offsets the cost savings of using them.)

When a device uses room air to assist in meeting the demands of the patient, it is considered a low-flow system. A low-flow system includes all systems we have listed for home use. Some things affect the level of oxygen available to you through low-flow systems. The following chart discusses a few of these as well as ways to troubleshoot them.

Troubleshooting Low Flow Circuit Chart

SYMPTOM	CAUSE	POSSIBLE SOLUTIONS
Soreness over ears or around nose/face	Irritation/ inflammation from tubing or straps	Loosen straps and place bandage, cotton ball, or foam between tubing/ straps and skin.
Mouth breathing	Blocked nasal passages	Use saline or nasal rinse to moisturize for easier expelling, or resort to simple mask if liter flow >5 lpm.
	Habitual mouth breathing	Complete breathing retraining exercises or resort to simple mask if liter flow >5 lpm.
No gas flow from cannula	Device not turned on	Go back to beginning; check that device is turned on and liter flow is correctly set.
	Leak in circuit	Check tubing for holes; replace tubing if necessary.
	Blockage or remove circuit	Check for kink in or blockage of hose; clear blockage or replace hose if damaged.
Humidifier pop off is sounding	Obstruction in circuit	Find and remove obstruction.
	Flow set too high	Use alternative device until flow setting is corrected.

Continuous Flow

CYLINDER SIZE	0.5 LPM	1 LPM	1.5 LPM	2 LPM	2.5 LPM	3 LPM	4 LPM	6 LPM	WEIGHT
M-4	3:46	1:53	1:15	0:56	0:45	0:37	0:28	0:18	2.6 lbs.
B	5:29	2:44	1:49	1:22	1:05	0:54	0:41	0:27	2.9 lbs.
C	8:16	4:08	2:45	2:04	1:39	1:22	1:02	0:41	4.4 lbs.
D	13:49	6:54	4:36	3:27	2:45	2:18	1:43	1:09	5.6 lbs.
E	22:44	11:22	7:34	5:41	4:32	3:47	2:50	1:53	8.0 lbs.
M-60	57:27	28:43	19:09	14:21	11:29	9:34	7:10	4:47	23.0 lbs.
M-M	115:04	57:32	38:21	28:46	23:00	19:10	14:23	9:35	40.7 lbs.

Conservation 3 to 1 Flow (based on 20 bpm)

CYLINDER SIZE	0.5 LPM	1 LPM	1.5 LPM	2 LPM	2.5 LPM	3 LPM	4 LPM	6 LPM	WEIGHT
M-4	11:19	5:39	3:46	2:49	2:15	1:53	1:24	0:56	2.6 lbs.
B	16:27	8:13	5:29	4:06	3:17	2:44	2:03	1:22	2.9 lbs.
C	24:50	12:25	8:16	6:12	4:58	4:08	3:06	2:04	4.4 lbs.
D	41:27	20:43	13:49	10:21	8:17	6:54	5:10	3:27	5.6 lbs.
E	68:13	34:06	22:44	17:03	13:38	11:22	8:31	5:41	8.0 lbs.

APPROXIMATE TANK TIME

The length of time an oxygen tank will last is dependent on the liter flow, conservation devices, if in use, and the size of the tank. Above are some approximate lasting times for different tank sizes and liter flows. This will help you determine how much time you will have on each tank and whether or not you need to take an extra tank as a backup for outings you will go on.

GET TO KNOW YOUR OXYGEN SUPPLIER

Be sure you talk with your oxygen supplier. Your supplier's job is to ensure you properly understand how your oxygen tanks, concentrator, and other equipment work. Don't be afraid to ask questions or ask for clarity of instructions or explanations your oxygen supplier gives. If you have a hard time receiving answers to your questions, call your physician's office.

Also, make sure you always have a backup supply of oxygen and other supplies in case of emergency.

OXYGEN STORAGE: SAFETY PRECAUTIONS

Oxygen itself is not flammable, but it does help any fire burn hotter and faster. Therefore, precautions need to be taken. Follow these safety tips:

- Let your local fire department know you have oxygen in your home, and always keep fire extinguishers (that are regularly maintained) in several rooms in your home. Make sure your address is easy to see from the street both day and night.
- If you have a concentrator in your home, make your power company is aware so they will give you higher priority during power failure.
- Keep stored tanks in a safe place where they won't tip over and get damaged. Any time tanks are stored in an enclosed space, the potential for leakage presents a fire hazard. It is best to store your tanks in a cart, standing and secured. Your tanks are heavy, and if they get knocked down, they can cause damage to property or hurt the person they fall on. Also, if the valve on the tank were to break off during a fall, the pressure could cause the tank to propel across the room, possibly through walls and definitely hurting anyone in its path. If you cannot store your tanks standing securely in a cart, store them lying down in a safe place where they will not be a trip hazard.
- Ensure tanks are stored in a well-ventilated area. Keep all oxygen supplies at least 10 feet away from any heat source. This includes any open flames (including candles), stoves (electrical or gas), countertop appliances that create heat (such as toaster ovens), electric hair dryers, clothes dryers (electric or gas), space heaters, furnaces, windows exposed to direct sunlight, radiators, etc.

- Do not allow smoking anywhere inside your home. See page 302 in the Appendix for a No Smoking sign that can be photocopied in multiple and placed by the entrances of your home and in any area where family members or visitors might forget and light up.
- It is also a good idea to put signs up alerting visitors that there is oxygen in your home. See page 301 in the Appendix for another sign to post, regarding your oxygen use and safety. Make several copies of it to place in windows by the entrances to your home, on your bedroom door, by the bed of the patient using oxygen, and where oxygen is stored. Make sure it is visible from at least a 5-foot distance.
- Avoid using flammable products around your oxygen. Do not use any petroleum-based products near your oxygen equipment, including your tubing and cannula. Use only water-soluble creams and makeup.
- Use fabric softeners to avoid static electricity buildup in your fabrics.
- Establish two escape routes from the home in case of fire. Practice using these routes. Keep a phone readily accessible to you from your bed (on the nightstand or a nearby table) in case you cannot escape, so you can call for help.
- If you live in a house with multiple levels, consider keeping a tank on each floor: I recently had a patient who stored an oxygen tank on the upstairs level of his home, and another in the basement bedroom of his home, so if he somehow got disconnected from his concentrator or had a break in his hose while he was in either of these locations, he would have adequate oxygen available to him for immediate attachment as opposed to struggling to get up or down the stairs and then resolve the problem while he was so short of oxygen. This is a perfect example of planning and putting safety first.

CPAP/BIPAP THERAPY

Many people need to use CPAP or BiPAP machines, as well as oxygen therapy, to help them get enough oxygen during sleeping hours and to help manage CO_2 levels in the late stage of COPD.

CPAP

CPAP (continuous positive airway pressure) is used at home to keep the airways open when you are sleeping. CPAP has one pressure setting that remains constant while running and is used to improve oxygenation—the amount of oxygen your body has made available to it.

Adherence to your CPAP treatment can be difficult, but it is important. Often, the most trying part of your treatment is adjusting to wearing the mask, which can be either a full-face mask (covering both your nose and your mouth) or a nasal mask (covering only your nose). It is a good idea to start out slowly when adjusting to your new mask. Wear it for a couple of hours a night, incrementally increasing your time until you are able to wear it all night. It is even a good idea to try wearing it awhile during your day to help you adjust to having it.

Don't be afraid to contact your supplier if you struggle too much wearing your mask. If you need to try a few different masks to find one that works for you, do so. Just be sure to ask your supplier what your insurance coverage is first, to avoid excessive expenses.

BiPAP

BiPAP (bilevel positive airway pressure) is similar to CPAP, but where CPAP has one pressure setting, BiPAP has two: a base setting and an inspiratory setting that gives you an additional burst of pressure when you inhale. BiPAP is used to help manage CO_2 levels and help with ventilation—the actual moving of air into and out of the lungs. This therapy is used at home by patients who retain CO_2 at levels that are considered too high by their physician. This CO_2 retention happens when air gets trapped in the air sacs and can't be expelled through normal breathing and when too much oxygen is used. This is usually first discovered when symptoms, such as headaches, drowsiness, confusion, lethargy, and sometimes a hand tremor, lead the patient to a doctor or hospital. To determine whether therapy is needed, the doctor has an

Jim's Story

Jim, a former patient of mine, has COPD and sleep apnea. Jim's wife was worried about his daytime drowsiness—and was complaining about his nighttime snoring!—so Jim's doctor ordered a sleep study.

For the study, electrodes were placed in various places on Jim's head, neck, and legs and an oximeter was used to monitor his blood oxygen levels. After he fell asleep, the electrodes recorded sleep patterns to determine what stage of sleep he was in and muscle movement in his legs as well as vibrations in his throat, which would indicate snoring, caused by an obstruction in the airway. As the techs watched him sleep, they saw his oxygen levels drop as low as 58 during certain periods of sleep. They then put a BiPAP on him, on the setting that best maintained his oxygenation and eliminated his snoring.

Although it took Jim a few weeks to get used to wearing the mask and breathing with the machine, he felt better when he woke up in the morning—and so did his wife! His daytime drowsiness improved, his snoring was eliminated, and his oxygen levels stayed in a safe range. And after he had been using his machine for a few months, his blood pressure was also reduced.

ABG drawn, showing exactly where the oxygen and CO_2 content are in the blood. The BiPAP machine helps hold the airways open and assists in moving air to help remove CO_2 from the alveoli. You can even use a simple mouthpiece, just like putting a straw in your mouth, as opposed to wearing a mask during your waking hours, to receive your BiPAP therapy and control your CO_2 levels. This is a wonderful new addition to therapy! How easy is it to hold a straw in your mouth and get assisted breaths? This is convenient because you won't have to bother with removing your mask if the phone rings, or someone comes to the door, or you would simply like to take a drink of your water (which should always be sitting beside you).

If You Have Sleep Apnea

You may use CPAP or BiPAP when you're asleep or awake. Both are used with patients who suffer from sleep apnea. There are a few types of sleep apnea, but the treatment for all can be the same. If you are using this to help regulate CO_2 levels in cases of chronic lung disease, you will most likely use this therapy during your waking hours, as well as sleeping.

In the most common form of sleep apnea, obstructive sleep apnea (OSA), the airways collapse when you relax. The pressure from the CPAP/BiPAP helps keep these airways open, so you can continue to breathe without as much interruption and waking. Your individualized setting for the device will be determined during a sleep study. You may or may not need to entrain extra oxygen into your line.

> ### Write It Down! My Oxygen Provider and Durable Medical Equipment Provider Information
>
> Turn to page 303 in the Appendix to record the information you may need in maintaining your oxygen and/or durable medical equipment, to have on hand for your own reference, your health-care providers, or in case of emergency.

Once you better understand the use of oxygen, including how it can improve your overall well-being, which devices are particularly useful toward remaining physically active or getting a good night's sleep, and how to properly store your oxygen supply, you will definitely find more success and fewer struggles in using it. Becoming familiar and comfortable with this form of assistance will help you breathe easier, both literally and figuratively. It is important for your fears to be alleviated. You will learn more on that in the next few pages.

Breathe Easier

Sometimes you wake up. Sometimes the fall kills you. And sometimes, when you fall, you fly.

—Neil Gaiman

Your stress levels directly impact your lung disease and your ability to breathe! This cycle of dyspnea (shortness of breath), referred to as the COPD Downward Spiral, is vicious: When you struggle to breathe, your stress level naturally rises, which makes it more difficult to breathe, which raises your stress level again, and so on.

But there *is* a way that you can naturally take charge of your breathing. When you learn controlled breathing techniques, you'll be able to manage your breathing rate and lessen the amount of energy it takes to breathe, while improving the position and condition of your respiratory muscles. Controlled breathing releases endorphins in your body, dilating blood vessels and increasing blood supply to the tissues. It lowers your blood pressure and heart rate and increases tissue oxygenation, allowing you to slow and control your breathing to a greater degree. It is another cycle, but this time it benefits you!

During controlled breathing, we strive to practice three things: pursed lip breathing, belly breathing (diaphragmatic breathing), and positioning. Practicing these things in a daily routine will help you in

Connie's Story

I worked with Connie in pulmonary rehab. She was in Stage 4 COPD with a strong asthma component. When she first came to rehab, even leaving her house gave her so much fear and anxiety, she often chose to stay at home. Over time this had a great impact upon her life and depression set in. Her anxiety would stem from embarrassment from wearing a nasal cannula on her face, fear of running out of oxygen, feelings of breathlessness when walking around, and difficulty and fatigue from pulling her oxygen tank with her. When her therapy first started, we would even go pick her up to bring her to therapy until she was ready to travel alone. We worked on managing her anxiety and dealing with her fears so she could once again take part in her life. A few weeks after therapy began she began to change. The transition was incredible to watch. She went from suffering from difficult anxiety attacks and not wanting to leave her home at all to helping other friends in her rehab group learn to deal with their own anxiety by following a few simple steps.

more ways than the ones listed above. Pursed lip breathing is essential for your recovery when you are feeling short of breath; belly breathing strengthens your respiratory muscles; and positioning will help you when you feel short of breath, are struggling with fatigue, or are just in need of a rest. Practicing these things daily will help them become second nature to you, so when you are in a tough situation or trying to recover, it will be natural for you to use these methods to help.

Controlling your breathing is the first step to help you relax. During the exercise portion of your pulmonary rehab program, you will be exercising your breathing muscles naturally as you increase the depth and rapidity of your breaths. Your primary breathing muscle is your diaphragm, which is the large muscle that separates your thoracic (chest) cavity and your abdominal (stomach) space. Although this is the strongest and primary breathing muscle, it is not the only one. We all have what are called accessory muscles, as well.

Our accessory muscles are found lining our rib cage, in our shoulders, and in our neck. These muscles help pull the chest wall up and out when we inhale and push it down and in when we exhale. Patients with chronic lung disease often use accessory muscles to breathe. Controlled breathing is one exercise we can do to strengthen these muscles.

BREATHING ESSENTIAL #1: PURSED LIP BREATHING

Pursed lip breathing is used to increase oxygenation when you feel stressed and short of breath, as well as during your meditation time (you'll learn more about meditation in Step 9, on page 235). The benefits of this are slowing the breathing pattern, enabling more stale air to be exhaled, and allowing more oxygenated air to enter the lungs for gas exchange.

Pursed lip breathing is accomplished by breathing at a ratio of one to two: one part in, two parts out. You breathe in for one to two seconds, and out for two to four seconds (the actual time is individual to each person). The name of this technique comes from the second part of the process: you breathe in through your nose, but out through pursed lips, as if you are blowing out a candle. A trick that might help you remember how to do pursed lip breathing is to imagine a birthday cake:

Smell the cake, blow out the candles: Inhale through your nose, exhale through your mouth.

The primary goal of pursed lip breathing is to create back pressure in your lungs. Recall that your lungs branch down from your throat, similar to the way a large tree branches upward toward the sky. The airways then branch out into smaller and smaller airways until they reach the alveoli, or air sacs, at the base of each branch. These tiny sacs stay open or close as a result of pressure changes within them. The great thing about pursed lip breathing is that when you blow out, as if you are slowly blowing out a candle, it builds back pressure in your airways, which allows the airways to stay open longer and more air to escape. When more air escapes, it, of course, needs to be replaced. What you will find is more available space in the air sacs for oxygenated

> Remember, if you feel short of breath . . .
> - Don't panic.
> - Perform pursed lip breathing.
> - You can do it!

air to enter when you inhale on your next breath. Although this method of breathing may feel unnatural, especially when you feel short of breath, it is ultimately a fantastic way to oxygenate yourself. You only need to do it when you are struggling for air, not all the time. Chances are, by switching to this method if you are straining to breathe, you will start to feel better in just a few breaths.

Because it is not the way you have spent your entire life breathing, it is important to practice it as often as you can, so you can swing into this technique comfortably whenever you need to.

Combining this practice with your relaxation time (see Step 4, page 115) will compound the benefits and save time and energy, exactly what we are trying to do! Practice this for at least fifteen minutes three times per day, and at least one of these times while you are resting after a meal or between activities.

BREATHING ESSENTIAL #2: BELLY BREATHING

Belly breathing, otherwise known as diaphragmatic breathing, is an exercise used to strengthen the breathing muscles. As with any other muscle in your body, the more these muscles are toned and used, the more efficient they will be.

To practice belly breathing, lie down or sit in a comfortable position in a recliner. Be in a position that allows your lungs to open as much as possible. If you can't lie back, practice good posture and sit up as straight as you can. Place one hand on your chest, and another on your stomach. What you will focus on during this exercise is taking nice, deep breaths that will come clear down to the bottom of your lungs and move your diaphragm, lifting the hand that is on your stomach with each breath while leaving the hand on your chest in a more steady position. Focusing on this activity will help you understand more clearly what a belly breath is and practice it for better oxygenation.

If you find it difficult to practice this with your hands placed on your chest and your stomach, try another method called the Butterfly (see page 108).

In general, whether one suffers from lung disease or not, most people tend to be rather shallow breathers. Shallow breathing uses the upper most portion of our lungs while leaving the air sacs of the lower portion unopened and unused. This limits the amount of oxygenation you give your body and also leaves the lower air sacs more susceptible to pneumonias, especially if you lead a more sedentary lifestyle.

Practice oxygenating yourself with belly breathing by doing three sets of ten breaths three times per day to start. In this exercise, you are using your abdominal and accessory muscles to move air. Squeeze them when you push the air out. Think of it as a push-up for your diaphragm. Listen to your body, and see how fatigued you get during this. You may get tired, even if you don't expect to. If you begin to feel dizzy or light-headed, rest. Use your pursed lips upon exhalation to prevent this.

Strengthen Your Diaphragm

When you have chronic lung disease, your diaphragm, which is normally dome-shaped, often becomes flattened over time. Your diaphragm moves to create the pressure difference that allows air to flow in and out of the air sacs in your lungs. When the pressure in your airways reaches a certain point, the airways collapse and no more air escapes. This leaves stale or used air trapped in the air sacs, taking up valuable space where fresh, oxygenated air should be. When the fresh, oxygenated air cannot move into your lungs, shortness of breath occurs.

Many times, you use accessory (secondary) muscles called intercostals to breathe. They are the muscles that line or surround your rib cage. The intercostals help you breathe when your diaphragm becomes less functional. By lifting the rib cage up and out as you inhale, they change the pressure in your airways. By pushing down and in, they push the air back out of your lungs when the time comes to exhale. Intercostals are a great support system, but your diaphragm is better.

Practicing using your diaphragm strengthens your normal breathing muscles. Belly (diaphragmatic) breathing increases proper breathing skills and strengthens your diaphragm, or natural breathing muscle. Using resistant devices when you practice your breathing enables you to exhale a greater amount of stale or used air, which leaves more room for new, oxygenated air to enter and allows your diaphragm to return to its more normal dome shape. Combining belly breathing with resistance, such as pursed lip breathing or using a device, such as a harmonica or your vocal cords, allows airways to remain open somewhat longer, enabling more stale air to escape from your air sacs. When this occurs, more oxygenated air can fill your air sacs and help relieve your shortness of breath.

Play the harmonica! Have you ever watched a harmonica player? If you have, you will remember the way their stomach moves with each breath. This is a great example of what strengthening your diaphragm should look like. When you practice your belly breathing, you are using the same muscle strengthening movements that harmonica players use. The harmonica also offers resistance and helps expel trapped air.

Sing! Another activity that strengthens your diaphragm is singing. If singing is something you enjoy doing, this is a great way to practice strengthening your breathing muscles and exhaling trapped air. When singing, you use your vocal cords. These create that back pressure in your airways that will enable you to let more stale or used air out of your air sacs. This leaves more room for new, oxygenated air to enter, supplying you with a fresh supply of oxygen, therefore reducing your shortness of breath.

BREATHING ESSENTIAL #3: POSITIONING YOUR BODY

When you are struggling to breathe, few physical positions will help open up your chest cavity and make it easier to breathe. All of these positions are thought to give the diaphragm more room to descend. It might not be a bad idea to try and practice these so they become more natural before you are in a situation where you feel short of breath and are working under distress. While in any of these positions, remember to practice your breathing techniques, especially pursed lip breathing, when you feel short of breath.

Positioning Tip #1: Standing

It is important to remember that good posture helps your breathing. Stand with your neck and back aligned, chin tucked under slightly, and buttocks tilted in slightly. This will open your trunk up so that your lungs can have optimal expansion. If you would like, you can try standing against a wall for this. It may help stabilize you and assist you in aligning yourself. If you struggle to pull your shoulders back, hold your arms down at your sides and turn your hands palm forward. This shifts your shoulders, opening up your chest and lungs.

You can stand leaning forward slightly, letting your arms hang slightly forward. This works well at home as well as in public when you may want to remain inconspicuous. An altered version of this position is to lean over with your hands resting on their upper thighs. When you do this, try using your shoulders and arms as a brace, further engaging your accessory muscles when you breathe. Some people like to alter this position by sliding their hands a little farther down their legs. Be careful not to place your hands beyond your knees, as this will actually make it more difficult to breathe, especially in people who have a pot belly.

A position similar to the one just described is to lean forward over an object that stands 3 to 4 feet tall. For many people a counter, table, or the back of a couch is the perfect height for this position. Lean forward, supporting yourself with your arms, allow your chest to open up, and practice pursed lip breathing. Try to relax, control your breathing, and calm yourself.

Positioning Tip #2: Sitting

Place your hands on your knees or thighs and lean slightly forward, bracing yourself, again, with your shoulders and arms. Once comfortable, relax, control your breathing, and calm yourself.

You can try leaning over the table, laying your head against your folded arms, opening up your chest, and allowing your diaphragm to descend. Practice pursed lip breathing. You can also use a pillow with this position, wrapping your arms around the pillow and raising it off the table. Relax, control your breathing, and calm yourself.

Positioning Tip #3: The Butterfly

Another sitting position is the butterfly. Sit up straight in a chair with your arms to your side and your feet flat on the floor. Place your hands behind your head and raise your elbows along with your shoulders. Breathe in slowly through your nose. As you breathe out slowly through pursed lips, bend slowly over toward your knees, bringing your elbows in toward your face. Bend over as far as is comfortable for you, and, as you inhale, raise yourself back up to your sitting position.

Positioning Tip #4: Lying Down

With COPD, it is a good idea to sleep with a few pillows supporting you. Many people find that the lower their head is, the more difficult it is to sleep. It is also important to listen to your body. If it is more difficult for you to breathe when lying down, especially if the problem is sudden or worsens over a few days, contact your physician.

One of the most comfortable positions is to lie on your side, your upper body supported by three or four pillows. Place another pillow in front of you to prevent you from slipping, and cross your top knee over in front of you. Relax, control your breathing, and calm yourself.

CONTROLLED COUGHING

Controlled coughing is a process that helps you remove the mucus from your lungs. It is accomplished in short sessions that enable you to expel, under controlled circumstances, the secretions that may be blocking your airways. You'll want to plan these sessions out when you have time to rest in between.

Coughing is nature's way of cleaning out the lungs. Our lungs make mucus to trap dirt and other particles that enter our lungs and help expel it. If this mucus is not expelled, it can leave us with a breeding ground for infection, cause blockages in our airways, shortness of breath, and wheezing. It is important to try and expel these secretions so this does not happen.

To perform a controlled cough, sit up in a chair, leaning slightly forward. Take a deep nasal breath, and hold it for 2 seconds. Bend forward and cough the first time to loosen the mucus. Cough again to move the mucus forward through the airway. Try not to inhale between the two coughs, as this could move the mucus back down the airway. When you perform these coughs, try not to make them large, but smaller and controlled. Use the diaphragm to push the air out, in a huffing motion— short and quick. After coughing twice, wait a few seconds and repeat the process over again. Inhale slowly and deeply. Inhaling quickly can push the mucus back down the airway. Repeat this process until you feel as if you have removed the mucus and don't have to cough anymore. Rest and relax. Be sure to spit coughed up mucus into a tissue and dispose of it.

POSTURAL DRAINAGE AND PERCUSSION

If you suffer from COPD or other lung diseases, you may very well be familiar with the mucus factory your lungs have become. Depending on how your mucus is, you may find it necessary and beneficial to use postural drainage and percussion therapy to help you move and cough up that gunk in your lungs.

There are a couple of different types of percussion therapy. Some methods may have a better effect on you than others.

Manual percussion: Your lungs are divided into lobes. The left lung is divided into two lobes, and the right is divided into three lobes. Each lobe has airways that lead back to the center of your chest so mucus can be removed. During manual percussion, your health-care provider will place you in different positions for each particular lobe that the percussion therapy is used for.

Once you're in the right position, your health-care provider will form his or her hands into a cupped shape and drum on your back, upper chest, or side. This cupping shape creates a pocket of air when the hands touch you. This air increases the amount of vibration the drumming causes inside the lungs, helping to dislodge mucus that is stuck against the airways, in the air sacs, or in pockets that have developed in the airways. With the mucus moving farther along in the airways, you will feel the sensation to cough. This is to be expected—don't let it alarm you. Be aware, however, that the coughing isn't always immediate. Sometimes it is up to hours later.

Another thing to be aware of is how your body feels during and after your percussion therapy. Your therapist or nurse should ask you during the therapy whether you are feeling okay, and whether the amount of pressure is comfortable. Let your provider know how you feel, and whether you would like him or her to drum with a little more or less force. Don't be nervous or afraid of having percussion therapy done. While it may sound intimidating to some, it is oftentimes relaxing and proves to be relieving and beneficial enough you may want it done again. Work with your therapist or nurse. Help him or her position your body into the poses that will enable the mucus to travel where it should so you can cough it up.

It would also be extremely beneficial to you to drink enough water. If you are on fluid restrictions from your physician, follow them explicitly. If you are not, increase your water intake to 8 to 16 glasses per day. This will thin the mucus in your lungs and make it less sticky and easier to mobilize. When it travels easier, you are going to cough more of it up.

Vest percussion therapy: Another form of percussion therapy can be found in the use of wearing a vest that is connected to a machine that fills the vest with air and then vibrates the air at adjustable frequencies and rates. There are various types of vests and the treatment can be done in various positions, from lying down to sitting up. It can be done for differing lengths of time and is often used in conjunction with a nebulized medication, which hydrates the mucus and causes it to loosen and move easier. This is another safe and effective method to remove the mucus in your lungs. Removing this mucus will increase the amount of space you have available for air movement and offer you more surface area for gas exchange. Resolving each of these issues will decrease your shortness of breath and help you feel better.

Be sure to use controlled coughing during and after your percussion therapy to remove the most mucus and gain the greatest benefit from it.

Learning these skills will help you in many ways, only one of which is energy conservation. At this point in your life managing your energy is essential to your well-being and your ability to function the best you can.

THE AIR YOU BREATHE

Does your home environment help or hinder your breathing? Have you switched your cleaning agent or detergent to products that do not have strong scents? Have you already removed air fresheners and candles from your home environment? Are you aware that those things not only feel irritating but they can actually cause your lungs to react in ways that can make breathing much more challenging for you, which is exactly what you don't want? Try to avoid the use of strongly scented cleaning agents, soaps, and detergents. Also avoid any products you need to spray to use, as the small particles from these can easily be inhaled and irritating.

If desired, you can replace harmful chemical cleaners with homemade vinegar solutions. Vinegar is a natural antiseptic and will kill many household germs. For use as a cleanser, add 2 cups of vinegar to 1 gallon of water (more or less according to personal preference), plus additional natural ingredients and essential oils, to create your own supply of fresh, nonirritating household cleaners for you (or whoever helps you clean) to use.

Following are my favorite, tried-and-true recipes for vinegar-based cleaners. For each recipe you can alter the amount of vinegar you add to your tap water according to your unique situation. The additional ingredients in these recipes will help the vinegar clean more effectively as well as smell better when used.

Remember to *never* reuse old cleaning agent bottles. *Only* use new containers for your homemade cleaners.

Orange Cleaner: Place your orange peels in a large canning jar and pour white vinegar over them. Let sit for a few days and the vinegar will adopt the scent of the oranges, leaving you with a fresh smelling, natural citrus base for your vinegar mixtures. You can also make a variation of this by adding lemon or lime peels to the mixture.

Floor Cleaner: Mix ¼ cup each of white vinegar and baking soda plus 1 tablespoon of dish soap to 2 gallons of hot water, for a natural, chemical-free floor cleaner. (This is where your citrus-blend vinegar can come in handy.)

Glass Cleaner: Use ¼ cup of vinegar to 2 cups of water for a nonirritating glass cleaner. Again, you can use your citrus blend, if you'd like. You can also add 1 tablespoon of dish soap for dirtier windows.

Carpet Cleaner: You can use a vinegar solution of 1:1 vinegar and water to clean your carpet. Spray or pour a small amount of the mixture on carpet stains and let it sit for a few minutes and then gently scrub the stain out with a clean scrubbing brush.

Straight vinegar is also an effective drain cleaner if you pour it directly into the drain and let it sit for 30 minutes, followed by flushing the drain with boiling water (get help for this job if you need it).

Vinegar aside, you can also utilize baking soda as a scrubbing agent (I use it all the time!) and regular, white toothpaste as a stain remover, to help avoid the strong scents and chemicals in many household cleansers.

Finally, I use olive oil plus 10 drops of lemon essential oil as my furniture polish. It is all natural, nonirritating, and leaves my wood with a beautiful shine.

Also, do your best to avoid strong chemical air fresheners in your car. It will probably be best for you to avoid scent all together in such a small space, but if you must, try mobile car diffusers for essential oils so you can avoid inhaling chemicals. These oils are safe to have around with your oxygen and usually nonirritating if used in small doses (you will usually add 2 to 3 drops to your diffuser and it should last quite some time).

Conserve Your Energy

You've done it before and you can do it now. See the positive possibilities. Redirect the substantial energy of your frustration and turn it into positive, effective, unstoppable determination.

—RALPH MARSTON

If you have lung disease, you have most likely had moments in which you have exerted yourself a little more than you could tolerate, or when you have felt extremely short of breath. As we've been saying all along (and as you probably know well in your own life), when you can't breathe, nothing else matters. Part of being a lung patient is learning to adjust to your new condition. Things you have done in the past with ease, without thinking, may need to be altered, including your method of doing everyday things, how you pace yourself, how well you plan your day, the way you prioritize things, and even the way you organize your home and life.

The COPD ABCDEs are easy guidelines to help you conserve energy, so you can more effectively accomplish the everyday tasks you need to do. We'll review them and see what we can change. Along with preserving your energy, it is very important that you take time to relax and meditate to help you reduce and manage stress, so that you can

Charlie's Story

When Charlie made it into the clinic that day, I could tell he was out of sorts. His shoulders slumped and he looked exhausted. I immediately pulled a chair out for him and he sat down with a thump. Placing the oximeter on his finger to check his heart rate (which was high) and oxygen levels (which were low), I turned up his oxygen until his sats reached the low 90s. When he could speak without struggling, I asked how he was. He said he was frustrated and stressed. His day had started out okay with morning meds, breakfast, and coffee. He had planned on running a couple of errands before coming to therapy, and that's where things got hard: He went to the post office, where he had to simply drop off a few letters to mail and buy some stamps. He struggled to get his oxygen tank out of the car because the car next to him pulled in too close to his door and he couldn't open it far enough. That made him use much more energy than he had planned, his saturations dropped, and he was very breathless. He had to lean against his car for a few minutes until he caught his breath. He finally made it into the post office and back to the car. Next, he stopped at the store to grab a few things where he was, again, met with additional struggles. This time, the automatic carts he usually used were all out, so he had to walk. He grabbed a regular cart but had trouble lifting his oxygen tank into it. When he finally got to the checkout line, it "took forever" to check him out. It made him tired to spend the extra energy walking and standing—he hadn't budgeted for that—and he still had to do therapy, drive home, and fix dinner. Charlie is really good at budgeting his energy and planning his schedule around what he can tolerate, but none of that worked today. He shook his head and asked whether he could rest a while longer before his exercises. After I helped him to a therapy bed to lie down for a little while, I reminded him that these things happen sometimes and that he was doing well. I recommended that he focus this time on meditating, listening to each breath he took, and work to throw away the negative thoughts because they make the anxiety worse, which makes his breathlessness worse and recovery slower. I turned on some soft music for him, turned off the lights, and shut the door to a crack. He focused on positive self-statements, accepting that his morning didn't go as he had planned, but that he could adapt and maintain a positive self-outlook for the rest of his day.

break the shortness of breath cycle that can progressively worsen your breathing. For this reason, I highly recommend that you focus a certain amount of time (during at least one of your rest periods daily) on the Four R's: relax, regenerate, rejuvenate, and revive.

THE COPD ABCDES FOR CONSERVING ENERGY

A Is for Aim

One key to managing a chronic ailment is to keep your focus. Striving to aim correctly will help you to be direct and purposeful. This helps eliminate any undue stress that can have a profound effect on you physically and emotionally. Stress can impair or slow you down significantly at times, which compounds your stress and affects your breathing.

An essential way to aim and keep your focus is to plan your schedule in advance; this can make a big difference in your exertion levels. Here are some tips:

Plan trips so you can make stops at stores or other locations in order of address. This uses your time more efficiently, helping you conserve your energy and use your oxygen wisely.

Spread out your obligations throughout the week. Do a little each day rather than loading up on one day.

Plan your most taxing activities around how you typically feel throughout the day. For example, if you have more energy in the afternoon, plan to do your errands then. If you have more energy in the morning, consider doing things then, such as prepping for meals to be eaten later in the day.

Organize your workspace and your home by placing the most-used items at arm or waist height. This will eliminate time and energy reaching for things or digging them out of cupboards or drawers. Examples include such things as toasters, microwaves, pans, and other commonly used kitchen items; towels, shavers, toiletries, and other personal items that are commonly used in the bathroom; and other things you frequently use such as books, computer, and so on. Also, keep a selection of your favorite, easy-to-don clothing on a clothes rack that is convenient to get to each day. This will make the task of dressing shorter, easier, and less taxing.

B Is for Bearings

Understanding where you are physically each day will help you determine which activities you can perform that day and what level of exertion you may be able to tolerate. It is important to not overdo it, to become familiar with what your "normal" is, and how you feel at different levels of activity. If you pay attention to your body and allow that mind-body connection to develop, you will soon be in a very good position to know quickly what your parameters are. Here are some pointers for getting your bearings about you:

> Decide how you feel and what you can tolerate this very moment, or this very day. Base your activities on your bearings.
>
> Be aware of your positioning and recovery time today (see page 106).
>
> Be aware of your posture. Keep your head and neck aligned and your chin slightly tucked. This opens your airway as much as possible. Keep your shoulders and hips in alignment.
>
> Pacing yourself throughout your daily activities will keep you feeling better.
>
> Don't rush to finish a task. SLOW DOWN. It is okay if you finish it tomorrow.
>
> Schedule rest periods throughout the day, including resting for 45 minutes after meals. Digestion takes a lot of oxygen, and it is okay for you to rest, especially if you have a large meal.
>
> Rest if you feel tired. Resting when you need to takes less time, overall, than it will to work to exhaustion and have to rest the entire following day.

C Is for Calculate

Everything must be done purposefully and with intent now, so it's going to help you tremendously to calculate your moves. Prioritizing your tasks will allow you to choose which ones are most important. Calculate the benefits and risks of each situation. Ask yourself whether it is wise for you to participate in a particular activity before you do so, and whether the benefits will outweigh the risks of performing that particular task. How do your "numbers" add up? This calculation is completely subjective; it's up to you—you get to decide. You are the only one who knows the answer to these questions. It is important for you to calculate what you want to do and what you have to do.

You may find that your role in your family, community, church, and so forth is changing as your needs change. Allow this to happen if this is the case. You are still an important part of your family and community, can still be happy, and with more realistic expectations you may find yourself more satisfied, as well.

Here are some tips on how to prioritize:

Decide which tasks are the most important to you. Delegate responsibilities to another person, if you can.

Alternate your tasks between difficult and less difficult ones.

Set limits. Make a responsible activity plan.

Use labor-saving techniques, such as soaking dishes before you wash them.

Use a basket or cart with wheels to hold and move things around the house.

Eliminate extra steps by wearing a terry cloth robe and slippers after your shower, to avoid having to dry off, and letting dishes air dry instead of towel drying them. Have a pair of slippers handy to step into from the shower.

Learn to let go of guilt. It is an unnecessary burden. Your task will still be there tomorrow if you are too tired to finish it now.

D Is for Decide to Be Deliberate

Decide what you can do. Only you know what you can do, so you need to be deliberate in how you perform. Be deliberate in how you breathe. Be deliberate in how you rest. Be deliberate in how you stand. How you move your body is instrumental in your lung and overall health. Small things can make a big difference, so keep these things in mind:

Move your feet when turning. This gives you a steady base for support and reduces falls and the risk of injury.

When you purchase footwear, look for shoes that are both safe and easy to put on. Some types of slip-on shoes are a great option.

Keep objects close to your body when lifting or carrying.

Try to keep your back straight when lifting something. Bend your legs instead. Conserve muscle use by tucking your buttocks in slightly, maintaining a pelvic tilt.

When standing, place one foot on a low stool.

When performing activities, exhale upon exertion and inhale upon rest.

E Is for Energy Conservation

Finally, E—here is a summary of the key energy conservation tips mentioned earlier as well as some additional simple, everyday reminders to help you keep a good store of energy.

Sit for as many activities as possible.

Lean on your arms for support.

Determine your best breathing time of day for activities.

Use a terry cloth robe to dry off after showering.

Use a shower chair so you can sit to shower.

When you cook, prepare extra food and freeze it for future use.

Use a cart for carrying several items, so only one trip is needed.

When doing daily chores, such as making the bed, do part of it, rest, and then continue with the remainder.

Plan ahead of time to avoid rushing.

Combine tasks to save time and energy when possible.

Don't try to do everything at once. Spread your tasks over hours, days, or the entire week.

RELAXATION

Relaxation now needs to be a vital part of your life, even if it has not been before. You are experiencing changes that can cause stress. Relaxation can help you deal with that stress in a more positive manner and help you manage it more effectively. Your mind and body both need relaxation exercises.

Relaxation isn't about spending time enjoying a hobby or having peace of mind. It is a process that decreases wear and tear on your mind and body and helps you enjoy a better quality of life. Many people find it difficult to relax. In many of us, there is this innate drive to keep going, to keep doing. At this point in your life, it is time to prioritize, decide what works best for you, and be deliberate about doing it. This is a priority, and the few minutes you take to do this will help you continue on throughout the day. The benefits of relaxation to your health and your well-being will help you accomplish more. The truth is you can't afford not to take this time for yourself. You can't afford not to relax. None of us can, really, but for you it is truer now than ever!

Relaxation has been shown to have the following positive effects:

- Slows your breathing rate, which reduces the need for oxygen
- Slows your heart rate, which gives your heart a rest
- Lowers your blood pressure
- Reduces anger and frustration, soothing emotions, which means less crying, irritability, anxiety, and frustration
- Improves your concentration for better problem-solving ability
- Reduces muscle tension and chronic pain
- Increases blood flow to the muscles
- Releases hormones dilating blood vessels for more effective blood flow

In addition to these benefits many people who practice relaxation report experiencing these outcomes:

- More energy

- Greater immunity to illness
- Greater efficiency
- Better sleep
- Increased concentration

Take short breaks often during your day. Give yourself room to simply "be" without the demands of "being" something to someone, even to yourself. As rest is the basis of activity, these restful periods will help you reset.

How to Relax

It is important to foster the mind-body connection within yourself. Listening to your body, quieting your mind, and taking care of yourself are more important now than ever before. Here is a simple exercise that will help you relax.

Begin by getting comfortable. The methods or positions we talked about a few pages back (pages 106–108) will help you do that. After you are comfortable, begin by steadying your breathing. If you need oxygen, be sure it is set on the correct setting before getting comfortable, so you don't have to interrupt your session. Close your eyes, and feel your body. Breathe in and out, steadily. Focus on just being. There are no expectations of you. There are no requirements of you. Just focus on being, on how you feel.

Notice the good feelings in your body. Concentrate on each element of those good feelings. Where are they? How do they feel? Now breathe. In and out: belly breathing in, pursed lip breathing out. In. Out. Repeat it over and over. Nice, deep breaths.

Notice the negative feelings in your body. Find areas of tension or stress and focus on them. Are your shoulders tight? How about your neck? Are your legs tired? How does your back feel? Breathe through the discomfort until you feel the tension and stress lessen. Let it decrease more and more with each breath. Then put it away. It doesn't belong here right now. Continue breathing. In through your nose, raising your belly as you breathe. Out through pursed lips, as long and slow as you can comfortably do.

Feel your heart rate slow. You are relaxing. Feel your breaths release your tension with each exhalation. Concentrate on your breathing. Concentrate on how it makes you feel, the rhythm and pace. Take time to become aware of all the details of the experience of breathing. It will comfort you to feel this natural rhythm, much like the rhythm of the ocean washing to shore. Continue to breathe, listening to your body, for at least 15 minutes. Shut out the rest of the world for this time. You deserve and need this time for yourself. It will allow you to rejuvenate, revive, and prepare for the rest of your day.

Stretching for Relaxation

When you finish your relaxation, before you get up and go about the rest of your day, take 2 minutes to stretch your muscles.

If you think back to when you were a child, stretching was a natural part of your day. How many infants do you see stretching when they wake up? How many children do you see do the same? As adults we sometimes condition ourselves to neglect these simple, yet essential movements. Muscle flexibility decreases with age. Stretching elongates those muscles, which will make performing daily tasks much easier.

With stretching, you can find relief from pain, increase your flexibility (which decreases injury), increase your energy levels, increase blood flow to various parts of your body, enhance your coordination, improve your posture (which will help your breathing), gain a greater range of motion of your joints, and create an overall greater sense of well-being.

Try these additional simple stretches each morning and see whether you find improvement in how you feel:

1. Start with your face: Tighten up the muscles of your face and then relax them. Open your jaw and stretch it out.

2. Sitting in a chair or on the side of your bed, roll your head from one side to the other slowly. Let it rest on each side for a few seconds and feel the stretch in your neck and over into your shoulders. Let your head fall forward and touch your chin to your chest for a few seconds and feel it stretch down into the base of your neck, then look up and feel the stretch through the front of your neck. Remember to breathe through these exercises, and stay within your limits. You will be able to do more each day if you are persistent.

3. From the same seated position, cross your left arm over the front of your chest and hold your elbow with your right hand. Pull it toward you slightly and leave it there for a few seconds. Repeat this with the other arm. Repeat this stretch on both sides one or two more times.

4. Now lift your legs slightly in front of you and move your toes up and down—toward you and then away. Repeat this stretch for a few minutes until you feel as if your legs have been stretched some. To increase difficulty in this exercise you can lift your legs higher, and even use a belt around the bottom of your leg to hold it in place and stretch it. If you would like to do this, simply hold each end of the belt in your hands, loop it around the bottom of your foot and lift your leg in front of you. Be sure you are sitting in a safe and stable place when you do this so you don't slip down out of your seat. You will feel the stretch in the back of your legs.

YOU HAVE THE POWER: POSITIVE SELF-STATEMENTS

Although COPD can make you feel helpless, it is important to remember that you can take control. You can actively prepare yourself for stressors and establish coping skills to deal with them. This will help you relax and reduce your anxiety. You may already have some sayings or mantras that you regularly use. If not, here are a few that might help.

When preparing for a stressor, think about these statements:

- "This may upset me, but I'll know what to do."
- "No negative self-statements. I'll just focus on what I can do."
- "Time for a few deep breaths. Relax and breathe."

When confronting and handling stress:

- "I can feel my stress alarm turning on, but that's normal for this situation. This tension can be my ally."
- "I know what I should do. I know what I can do. I am okay."
- "It's too bad this is happening, but it's not a catastrophe. I'll survive and be just fine."
- "Don't make more out of this than you have to. Stay calm, just relax."

> **Write It Down!**
> **My Relaxation Record**
>
> Take a few minutes to keep track of the days you stretch in the chart on page 304 in the Appendix.

When coping with feeling overwhelmed:

- "I'll probably think this is funny later."
- "It's okay to give my attention to only one thing at a time instead of multitasking."
- "Just for today. One day at a time. I got through yesterday; I'll make it through today."
- "When this is over, I'm going to take a well-deserved rest."

Rewards for coping:

- "That could have been a lot worse. I actually got through that pretty well."
- "Wait until I tell so-and-so about this!"
- "I guess I've been getting upset for too long when it really wasn't necessary."
- "Now I know I can handle it if this ever happens again."

Positive attitude, relaxation, and the other elements discussed in this chapter can be life changing when implemented and used consistently. I've seen it happen time and time again! Learning to manage your medications is also important. Preventing flare-ups is one of your highest priorities! Read on to learn how.

Prevent Flare-Ups: Use Your Meds Effectively

Always laugh when you can. It is cheap medicine.

—LORD BYRON

Understanding your symptoms is vital to your disease management—and you'll be prescribed medications to help control your symptoms. Medications are an integral part of controlling your lung disease. Managing your disease effectively will help you keep your airways expanded and prevent blockages and exacerbations. A perfect example of this is my patient and dear friend Jan.

Jan was in the advanced stages of COPD and was struggling with keeping her breathing under control. She was kind of stuck in a tough spot where, because of recent progression of her disease, her medications needed to be reevaluated and her course of care had to be revisited. She worked very, very hard at therapy and did everything else she could to manage her disease. The amazing thing about Jan is that even through extra struggles such as these, she always had a contagious smile on her face and a laugh that you couldn't help but share. Jan knew her stuff. She monitored everything about her condition, so when she felt things starting to slip, it didn't take long before she brought it, not only to my attention, but to her pulmonologist's attention as well. She knew something wasn't right. Well, it took close to a year to get the right combination of medications determined and some of her medications were changed more than once, but after making those adjustments—a huge part of this continuing on was Jan's continued self-advocacy—Jan finally came out on top with medications that helped manage this new stage of her disease in a much more effective way. She always says, "I do my neb 'n' meds first; they're more important than any phone call or visitor or anything else. That's what keeps me on track."

A COPD exacerbation, or flare-up, is an increase or new onset of more than one COPD symptom, such as cough, mucus, shortness of breath, and wheezing that requires medicine beyond your rescue medication. If you experience an exacerbation, new medications may be added temporarily to the list of those you use regularly. These will help alleviate and control your symptoms.

Your physician will be the one to determine which medications are best for you, depending on the combination and severity of the conditions you have. Medications for the control of asthma, for instance, may be different than those used to control differing levels of COPD. Don't be afraid to ask questions!

Be sure to use your prescribed medications as directed and promptly report any problems or issues to your physician. It is a good idea to bring a list of your medications with you to all appointments you have. It is also smart to have your physician help you determine what other therapies will help you manage your lung disease and establish lifestyle modifications that will enable you to experience fewer symptoms and more good days. You now have many options to assist you in gaining control of your condition. While your physician plays an important role in your care, the things you do at home are even more important. Remember, YOU are the most important member of your health-care team.

Some things to consider/ask your physician are as follows:

- How many cups of water should I drink in a day?
- What are my medications, and when is the proper time and method to take them?
- What delivery method do my medications require? How much time do I need to take them?
- Are there any side effects to my medications?
- What can I do to decrease my symptoms?
- What over-the-counter meds, supplements, or foods may interact negatively with my medications?
- What should I do if I miss a dose?

TYPES OF MEDICATIONS

To properly manage your medications, your doctors and pharmacists need your help. Keep an up-to-date list of all your medications (these include any over-the-counter products, such as analgesics, as well as supplements and herbs) in your purse or wallet at all times. Take it with you to all of your appointments. It can help your providers greatly. For most lung disease symptoms, you will have a controller medication and a rescue medication. We will review both in the next few pages.

If you suffer from asthma, the most important controller medication you will take will be an inhaled corticosteroid. If you suffer from COPD, the most important controller medication you will have will be

Write It Down! My Pharmacies

It is a great idea to have the name and number of your pharmacist handy for when questions arise. You can use the chart on page 289 in the Appendix. In some situations, pharmacists can answer medication questions better than your physician or nurse. Make an effort to use the same pharmacy to fill all of your prescriptions, and check that your records at that pharmacy include a list of not only your drug allergies but also any food or drug allergies that you have. This way, your pharmacist can help you watch for interactions and advise you in a more effective manner.

a long-acting bronchodilator. If you have severe COPD, you will most likely be prescribed oxygen therapy, as well. When a single controller medication fails to effectively manage your symptoms, your physician will most likely prescribe you a combination medication consisting of an inhaled corticosteroid, long-acting bronchodilators, anticholinergics, and even xanthines. Fortunately, many of these therapies are now combined into one dose, making it easier for you to manage your medications and remain adherent (very important), especially when symptoms are no longer evident. Now, let's move on and review the different types of medications that are available.

Bronchodilators: Airway Openers

If you have COPD, you are probably familiar with the term *bronchodilator*. But if not, let's review it. Bronchodilators are airway openers: They help dilate your airways, making them larger. This allows air to travel through the airways more easily and effectively, improving oxygenation and gas exchange. These medications are typically used in conditions of reversible airflow obstruction, such as acute and chronic bronchitis, emphysema, bronchiectasis, cystic fibrosis, and other obstructive states.

Bronchodilators can be taken orally (through your mouth) or through an aerosol (inhaler or nebulizer). Some bronchodilators are short-acting. This means they will act quickly and are safe to use for emergency episodes. Short-acting medications are often termed rescue medications.

Other bronchodilators are referred to as long-acting or maintenance bronchodilators. These are prescribed for daily use and help you maintain an open airway. Most patients are prescribed both long-acting and short-acting medication.

Number One Rule

If you have a rescue medication, keep it with you always! Do not leave home without your rescue medications!

It is important to use these medications as prescribed. It is also important to use them in the correct order. If you have a steroid inhaler, too, use the

Rescue Medications vs. Maintenance Medications: What's the Difference?

Rescue medications are those that are short-acting (they go to work quickly) and are safe to use during an emergency. Your physician will let you know which medications are your rescue meds. Always keep your rescue medication with you at all times.

Maintenance medications are taken on a regular basis, at either 12- or 24-hour intervals. These medications are not used in emergency situations, and you may not recognize the benefits of taking them immediately. They take anywhere from four days to two weeks to build in your system and help control your symptoms on a long-term basis.

bronchodilator first, followed by the steroid. Using them in this order will open up your airways and allow the steroid to penetrate deeper into the lungs. Be sure to rinse your mouth following the use of an inhaled steroid. (Read more about the use of inhaled steroids on page 135.) You may also be prescribed xanthines (see page 134), which work by relaxing the smooth muscle surrounding the air passages of the lungs allowing them to widen and air to flow.

Some potential side effects of bronchodilators are:

- Increased heart rate
- Nervousness
- Headache
- Insomnia
- Shakiness
- Tremor
- Bad taste in mouth

Note all side effects that you have experienced and be sure to tell your physician about them.

It is important to remember that a tolerance to these medications will usually occur, lessening any side effects over time, but if you feel any of these side effects, you should contact your physician. If you take your bronchodilators as oral medication, remember to only take these medications as your physician prescribes.

Bronchodilator Modes of Delivery

Bronchodilators work in different ways, or use different paths to get to their destination. Think of it as having the choice of walking through the front door of your house, the back door, or a side door. All three doors will get you into your house, but each gives you a different route to take. Similarly, bronchodilators have different paths of delivery.

BETA-AGONISTS

Beta-agonists can be taken orally or through inhalation. There are basically two types of beta-agonist inhalers: quick acting and long acting.

Quick-acting beta-agonists include your rescue medications. These medications relieve shortness of breath quickly (usually within a few minutes) and should always be with you. They include the following:

Quick-Acting Beta-Agonists

MEDICATION	DURATION
Albuterol (Ventolin, Proventil)	4–6 hrs.
Levalbuterol	6–8 hrs.
Fenoterol	4–6 hrs.
Terbutaline	4–6 hrs.

Long-acting beta-agonists: Long-acting beta-agonists relax the muscle bands that surround the airways and allow you to breathe in and out more easily. **Long-acting beta-agonists are not rescue medicines** and do not relieve sudden symptoms. These are used to control symptoms for hours (12) at a time and should be used regularly whether you feel symptomatic or not.

They include the following:

Long-Acting Beta-Agonists

MEDICATION	DURATION
Formoterol	12+ hrs.
Salmeterol	12+ hrs.
Serevent	12+ hrs.
Symbicort	12+ hrs.
Foradil	12 hrs.
Indacaterol	24 hrs.
Umeclidinium/vilanterol combination (Anoro)	24 hrs.
Aformoterol (Brovana)	12 hrs.

ANTICHOLINERGICS

An anticholinergic is not used for fast relief, either. It is a slow-acting bronchodilator. **This does not replace your rescue medication.** Anticholinergics inhibit the transmission of parasympathetic nerve impulses and thereby reduce spasms of smooth muscle, such as the muscle lining your airways. The most common anticholinergics for airway control are in the following tables.

Short-Acting Anticholinergics

MEDICATION	DURATION
Ipratropium bromide (Atrovent, Apovent, Aerovent)	6–8 hrs.
Oxitropium bromide (Oxivent, Tersigen)	7–9 hrs.

Long-Acting Anticholinergics

MEDICATION	DURATION
Tiotropium bromide (Spiriva)	24 hrs.
Aclidinium bromide (Tudorza Pressair)	12 hrs.
Umeclidimium (Incruse Ellipta)	24 hrs.

Combination Drug Therapies

Some products combine a beta-agonist with an anticholinergic. They include:

Short-Acting Beta-Agonist Plus Anticholinergic in One

MEDICATION	DURATION
Fenoterol/ipratropium (Berodual)	6–8 hrs.
Albuterol/ipratropium (DuoNeb)	6–8 hrs.
Albuterol/ipratropium (Combivent)	6 hrs

Respimat inhalers: These inhalers deliver the medication by combining a traditional inhaler style with a nebulizer-style mist. It is an effective delivery method for most people and for those who have a hard time inhaling forcefully enough for dry powder inhalers and timing the use of metered-dose inhalers (see page 143 for more about these). Medications currently available in this delivery method include:

Respimat Inhalers

MEDICATION	DURATION
Respimat Spiriva	24 hrs.
Combivent Respimat	4 hrs.
Striverdi Respimat	24 hrs.

Liquid medications: Xanthines are a group of orally administered chemicals that include caffeine, dyphilline, guaifenesin, theophylline, and theobromine, which cause stimulation to the central nervous system, stimulate cardiac muscle, relax smooth muscle, improve contraction of the diaphragm, and encourage diuresis of the kidneys.

Anti-Inflammatory Medications

Inflammation is a protective response tissues have as a result of injury or irritation. When you feel short of breath, sometimes inflammation of the airway is part of the reason. Sometimes the mucus production is a result of the swelling of the tissues lining the airways. For this purpose, anti-inflammatory drugs are sometimes prescribed to reduce your symptoms. **These drugs are not rescue breathers. They DO NOT give immediate relief**, but once taken regularly, they can reduce the swelling and mucus production and offer you some relief from your symptoms.

Anti-inflammatory drugs can come in several forms. The important thing to remember with these drugs is to **never change, alter, or stop your dosage without speaking with your doctor first**. Anti-inflammatory medications can be either steroidal or nonsteroidal. Aerosol or liquid anti-inflammatories can be inhaled orally or nasally. They also come in pills or are administered by injection,

These drugs have possible side effects. Report any side effects to your physician.

- Sore throat
- Hoarseness
- Cough
- Bloody or black stools
- Unusual tiredness/weakness
- Weight gain

- Stomach discomfort
- Burning in stomach
- Stomach pain
- Back or rib pain
- Swelling in lower legs
- Mood swings

Oral Inhalation Steroidal Anti-Inflammatory

Oral steroidal therapy is usually prescribed as an anti-inflammatory maintenance therapy for mild to moderate persistent asthma and some cases of COPD. Oral steroids affect your body systemically, thus serving their purpose of helping your airways. Another way to assist in the reduction of inflammation and swelling in your airways is through inhaled steroids.

Steroid inhalers are used to reduce inflammation, swelling, and mucus production often associated with asthma and COPD. They act directly at the site in managing your inflammation; a good way to avoid some of the systemic side effects of steroids is to take them through an inhaler, localizing their effect to the lung tissue. You are more likely to be prescribed a steroid inhaler if asthma is part of your COPD diagnosis. If you are using orally inhaled steroids, it is important to remember that you should:

Use them secondary to using your bronchodilator. Allow 15 to 20 minutes between taking your inhaled bronchodilator and your inhaled steroidal medication. This will allow the airways to open up, and the steroid medication can reach farther into the lungs.

Always rinse your mouth after using your inhaled steroid. The use of inhaled steroids can sometimes increase the likelihood or risk of developing thrush. Thrush, also called oral candidiasis, is caused by an overgrowth of the yeast in the mouth. This happens because of a decrease in the infection-fighting ability of the immune system in the mouth as a result of using inhaled steroids. Thrush can normally be prevented with mouth rinsing and tooth brushing after the use of inhaled steroids, but some people tend to get thrush despite taking measures to prevent it. Your doctor will be able to help you if this happens.

Finally, it will take about three weeks for your steroid inhaler to reach its full potential and work completely, and although the usual side effects of oral medications or shots of steroids do not generally occur with inhaled steroids, some people do experience some of the following side effects:

- Sore throat
- Cough
- Hoarseness

If these persist, contact your physician.

Inhaled Corticosteroids

INHALED CORTICOSTEROIDS .
Beclomethasone dipropionate
Triamcinolone acetonide
Flunisolide
Fluticasone propionate
Budesonide
Fluticasone propionate/salmeterol
Mometasone
QVAR
Azmacort
AeroBid, AeroBid-M
Flovent, Flovent rotadisk
Pulmicort
Advair

COMBINATION INHALED CORTICOSTEROID AND LONG-ACTING BETA-AGONIST	DURATION
Fluticasone Furoate/Vilanterol (Breo Ellipta)	24 hrs.
Mometasone Furoate/Formoterol (Dulera)	12 hrs.

Intranasal Steroids

Intranasal steroids are used for the control of seasonal allergic or non-allergic rhinitis. Anti-inflammatory medications reduce inflammation in the walls of your airways, making the airways larger. This allows for more airflow and better oxygenation.

Oral Steroids

It's very important to obey your instructions when you are taking steroids orally (typically in pill form). You need to be aware of the following:

- Make sure all your doctors know you are taking them.
- Watch for such symptoms as stomach discomfort, burning, or pain after taking a steroid.
- Take them on schedule, at the same time every day.
- Take them after a meal. Some people like to do it right after breakfast, as taking them in the evening can interfere with sleep. If you cannot take them with food, drink milk or another antacid liquid.
- **Never** stop taking them without consulting your doctor, and be sure to inform your doctor that you are taking them before any surgeries (yes, even dental surgeries).

Daliresp

Daliresp is the brand name of a new prescription drug, roflumilast, which is a phosphodiesterase 4 inhibitor. Used in cases of severe COPD to reduce the number of exacerbations, it is an oral medication taken once daily to reduce inflammation in the airways of the lungs. It is different than any of the other medications available right now.

Up until the release of this medication, the only type of medications used to treat the inflammation in the airways had been steroids. The problem with steroids is that they are nonselective to particular cells. Roflumilast targets specific cells and thus reduces the inflammation in the airways more effectively.

It is important to remember that **Daliresp is not a rescue medication** (not a bronchodilator). **It is not to be taken in the event of an emergency and should not be used to treat sudden breathing problems.** It is intended to be used once daily, as a maintenance-type medication, and may reduce the number of exacerbations you will experience.

As with any drug, it carries with it side effects. Some are worse than others, but all should be noted. As listed from the drug information provided from the makers of the drug, Daliresp may cause the following:

Mental health problems, including suicidal thoughts and behavior: Some people may experience mood or behavior problems, including thoughts of suicide or dying, attempts of suicide, trouble sleeping, new or worsened anxiety, new or worsening depressions, acting on dangerous impulses, and unusual changes in behavior or mood. Be sure to tell your health-care provider if you have a history of mental health problems, including depression and suicidal behavior.

Weight loss: If you take this drug, you should check your weight on a regular basis. Your health-care provider will want to check your weight regularly. If you notice that you are losing weight, contact your health-care provider. It may be necessary to stop taking this drug if you lose too much weight.

Drug interaction effects: Daliresp may affect how other medications work, and other medications may affect how this drug works. Be sure to have your list of medications with you when you go to your medical appointments, so your health-care provider has a clear understanding of all prescription and nonprescription drugs you are taking. This includes any and all herbal supplements and vitamins.

Liver problems: You should not take Daliresp if you have certain liver problems. Talk to your health-care provider if you have a history of liver problems.

Other, less serious side effects include:

- Diarrhea
- Back pain
- Decreased appetite
- Nausea
- Flu-like symptoms
- Headache
- Dizziness

Remember, of course, you may have individualized side effects that may not be listed here. If you experience any of the above-listed effects or any other persistent, bothersome symptoms that do not go away, report them to your health-care provider. Your pharmacist can also provide you with more information on this, as well as on any other drug you are prescribed. Do not hesitate to use their fountain of knowledge. If you are pregnant or breastfeeding, please let your physician know. It may not be advisable to take this drug, as the passing of it through breast milk and harm to the unborn child are currently unknown. Most important, take Daliresp exactly as prescribed by your physician, follow all instructions included in the drug enclosure, let your physician know of any side effects, and listen to your body. Remember your mind-body connection—you are working on becoming acutely aware of your normal and listening for anything that deviates from that.

Nonsteroidal Anti-Inflammatories

These drugs are a growing class of medications for the preventive treatment of mild, persistent asthma. Some examples of nonsteroidal anti-inflammatory medications are the following:

- Zafirlucast (Accolate)
- Montelukast (Singulair)
- Zileuton (Zyflo)

Antibiotics

Antibiotics include:

- Azithromycin
- Clarithromycin
- Erythromycin
- Tetracyclines (Doxycycline)
- Fluoroquinolones (gemifloxacin, levofloxacin, moxifloxacin)
- Cephalosporins (Ceftriaxone, Cefotaxime, Cefepime)
- Penicillin (Amoxicillin, Ampicillin)
- Vancomycin

These drugs help fight infections in the body. Infections in the lungs can cause excess mucus secretion and swelling—which in turn can cause blockages in our airways and reduced oxygenation. It is important to understand that antibiotics will help your body fight bacterial infections, but they will not help you with viral infections, such as colds. At the time of your office visit your provider will use cultures of your body fluids and/or blood as well as signs and symptoms you are suffering to determine whether an antibiotic will be beneficial to you.

Antibiotics can also create a range of possible side effects. Report any side effects to your physician.

- Nausea
- Vomiting
- Diarrhea
- Rash
- Hives
- Headache
- Insomnia
- Stomach upset

- Indigestion
- Dry mouth
- Itching
- Irritation
- Restlessness
- Fatigue
- Yeast infection

Cough Medications

Cough medications help move the blockages out of your airways so you can oxygenate better. It is unusual for a physician to prescribe cough suppressants for those diagnosed with COPD, to treat the COPD. You may be prescribed one for a secondary, temporary condition, such as a viral illness. Never take any over-the-counter (OTC) cough medications without first consulting your physician. If you experience any side effects, such as those listed here or others, call your physician or pharmacist.

These are many possible side effects of cough medications. Report any side effects to your physician.

- Drowsiness
- Dry mouth
- Dizziness
- Fatigue
- Headache

- Dry eyes
- Nausea
- Diarrhea
- Decreased respiratory secretions
- Urinary retention

Mucus-Controlling Agents

Use your bronchodilator therapy prior to using your mucus-controlling agents.

Mucus-controlling agents are used to reduce the amount of airway secretions, with improvement in lung function and gas exchange. They also help with prevention of recurrent respiratory infections and consequent airway damage. Diseases that these medications are typically used for include those with excessive mucus production, such as COPD, tracheobronchitis, and bronchiectasis.

Mucus-controlling agents include the following:

- Acetylcysteine (10% or 20% solution)
- Dornase alfa
- Aqueous aerosols (water, saline)

Here are the possible side effects of mucus-controlling agents. Report any side effects to your physician.

- Bronchospasm
- Disagreeable odor
- Runny nose
- Voice change
- Chest pain
- Airway obstruction
- Nausea
- Sore throat
- Rash
- Conjunctivitis

Be sure to read the section on controlled coughing (Step 3, page 109). Controlled coughing is a technique often used in conjunction with mucus-controlling medications and is very effective in helping you expel the mucus in your lungs.

Inhaled Anti-Infective Agents

People who have some chronic lung conditions or suffer from immuno-compromised conditions, such as HIV, may be prescribed anti-infective agents. If this applies to you, it will be addressed individually and specifically depending on which agent you are presently taking and questions or concerns you may have. Anti-infective agents include the following:

- Pentamidine isethionate (NebuPent)
- Zanamivir (Relenza)

- Ribavirin
- Tobramycin (Tobi)

These drugs have many side effects. Report any side effects to your physician.

- Skin rash
- Conjunctivitis
- Bronchospasm
- Diarrhea
- Vomiting
- Sinusitis
- Headaches

- Red eyelids
- Loss of hearing
- Cough
- Nausea
- Bronchitis
- Dizziness

Inhaled Anti-Infective Agents

Three types of devices are used for inhalation medications:

Metered-dose inhalers

Dry powder inhalers

Nebulizers

Each of these are used completely differently, so it is crucial that you know how to use your device in order to receive your proper medication dosages. Each of these devices will be reviewed in depth for your understanding. Be sure to keep track of any questions you may have for your health-care provider.

Metered-Dose Inhalers

What's great about using a metered-dose inhaler (MDI) is that they are compact, portable, easy to use, and go into effect in a short amount of time. But there can be a few disadvantages to using an MDI. One is that it requires more hand-breath coordination than do other types of inhalers. This is eased with the use of a spacer device—an extension tube that fits between the inhaler and you. This looks similar to a toilet paper tube. MDIs used without a spacer can deposit some of the medication into your mouth, rather than fully down your airway; however, the use of a spacer will help prevent this from occurring. Another downside of MDIs is that they require you to hold your breath for a specified length of time, to ensure optimal medication delivery; this may be difficult for you to do consistently. Finally, it is also possible to make some errors while using your MDI. Common mistakes include assembling the device incorrectly, failing to remove the cap before actuation (squeezing the top of the inhaler down to deliver the medication), inhaling too quickly, accidentally actuating multiple times per dose into your "chamber" or other reservoir prior to inhaling, and waiting too long after actuation to inhale the medication from your MDI.

With MDIs, there is not generally any "counter" to track your doses. The typical MDI holds between 120 and 200 doses, depending on the amount of medication dispensed and propellant used in each dose. Each MDI will indicate specifically how many doses it holds. Once you reach the actuation number indicated on the canister, the percentage of medication in each dose will decrease. If the amount of medication in each dose decreases, your treatment will not be as effective, and this can be dangerous.

You can track the number of days your inhaler will last by dividing the amount of dosages you are prescribed to use daily by the number of dosages in the device. (For example, Flovent has 120 actuations. If you take four doses per day, it will last for thirty days.) Mark on your calendar the day your device should run out of medication, as well as the day one week prior to that, to alert you to refill your prescription.

Various propellants are used with MDIs. If you change medications and notice a difference in taste, that you need to prime the MDI, a different "speed" at which the medication leaves the inhaler, a different temperature of the medication upon delivery, or a new instruction for holding or not holding your breath after each actuation, it most likely has more to do with the propellant used as opposed to the actual medication. Be sure to continue to use your medication as prescribed, even if you feel a change, until you talk to your health-care provider. Chances are that you are still receiving the correct dose of medication.

HOW TO USE AN MDI

It is important to use a spacer or AeroChamber with your metered dose inhaler. If you do not have one, ask your physician to prescribe you one.

An AeroChamber is a holding chamber that contains a one-way inspiratory valve to hold the aerosol until you inhale it. Both devices attach to the end of the inhaler, allowing the large particles in the spray to settle on its walls. This provides a greater opportunity for the finer particles of medication to travel to the deepest parts of your lungs. This method of delivery is markedly more effective than the use of a metered-dose inhaler without a chamber. Measurement of medication delivery has shown to be up to 40 percent more effective with use of a spacer or chamber, meaning you will receive a truer delivery of your prescribed dosage of medication.

If you receive a plastic device, there is a good chance it will hold a strong static charge when it is new. You should wash this device in warm, soapy water and allow it to air dry prior to use, so as not to interrupt the delivery of medications.

Also, if you are prescribed more than one dose of your inhaler, take the first dose, wait a few minutes, and then take the second dose. The first dose will serve to open up your airways, allowing the second dose to get deeper into your lungs.

Follow these steps to use your MDI:

1. Remove the cap from the end of the MDI; inspect for debris or blockages.
2. Shake the MDI in preparation for actuation. If not used within a specific time, discharge one dose to prime the valve.
3. Exhale a normal exhalation.
4. Hold MDI on lower teeth (if you do not have a chamber), flatten your tongue, and seal your lips around the mouthpiece on either your chamber or your inhaler.

5. Begin to inhale slowly and then actuate the MDI simultaneously (your inhalation should take 3 to 4 seconds).

6. Continue to inhale to total lung capacity, hold your breath for 10 counts (seconds), and exhale normally.

7. Repeat these steps, as prescribed, for additional doses. Wait 30 seconds between each dose. Clean your actuator (the case your inhaler comes with) whenever you see buildup, or crusty residue, on it. To clean it, rinse it in warm water for 30 to 45 seconds, using a cotton swab to clean the inside of it. Shake off any excess water (do not wipe the device), and let it air dry overnight. If the actuator is not cleaned periodically, you can lose up to 30 percent of your medication delivery with each actuation.

Dry Powder Inhalers

As with MDIs, there are advantages and disadvantages to using a dry powder inhaler (DPI). Your physician can help you decide which delivery device is best for you. The advantages of using a DPI are that they are small and portable and, unlike the MDIs, come with a built-in dose counter. They are breath actuated and require a short preparation and administration time. The disadvantages are that the ability to properly use this device is dependent upon your ability to suck in air with sufficient speed and force. (Your physician should be able to measure whether you have the inhalation strength to use a dry powder inhaler.) You are also generally less aware of the delivered dose because it is so small, and it is somewhat susceptible to humidity, so these devices need to be stored in a cool, dry place. The soft part on the top of your mouth as well as the back of your throat can be impacted by the use of medications in this device, so be sure to follow the instructions recommended by the manufacturer and pharmacist regarding your prescribed medication.

Here are some common errors that can cause complications with a DPI:

- **Improper positioning:** It is important to keep the device in the appropriate position. Not doing so may allow the powder to fall out of the device, thus reducing your dose.
- **Exhaling into the device:** This can dampen the powder, interrupting the delivery of the medication by either causing it to clump or losing powder, both of which will reduce the dose. The humidity issue is also one to consider when deciding where to use it. A steamy bathroom will have the same effect upon the powder as exhaling into it.

There are four different types of dry powder inhalers, sold under the brand names Aerolizer, Diskus, Flexhaler, and the Asmanex Twisthaler. If you use one, please read the following general instructions.

HOW TO USE AN AEROLIZER (DPI)

If you use an Aerolizer, your medication requires you to remove a capsule from a blister pack and place it in the device for inhalation. Be sure to wait to remove the capsule from the blister pack until immediately before your prescribed dosage time. Also, be careful not to exhale into the device. This can displace powder and add humidity to it. The humidity can cause the powder to be damp and possibly clump.

To use your Aerolizer, perform the following steps:
1. Hold device upright.
2. Carefully place the capsule in the chamber of the device, not directly into the mouthpiece. As you squeeze the button(s) to puncture the capsule, listen for a click indicating that the capsule has been punctured. Feel for a vibration when you inhale. (You want the vibration to occur. No vibration can mean that the capsule may have come unseated in the chamber.)
3. Exhale, through pursed lips, until your lungs are completely empty.
4. Tip your head slightly backward.
5. Put your mouth around the opening, carefully angling it so the powder does not fall out.
6. Suck in as quickly and deeply as you can.

7. Hold the powder in your lungs for 10 seconds.

8. Remove the device from your mouth and turn your head away from the device to exhale. (Remember, you do not want the inside of the device to get damp from exhalation.)

9. Open the device and check that the capsule is empty. If any powder remains, close the device, return to step 1, and repeat, this time without inserting another capsule into the device.

HOW TO USE A DISKUS (DPI)

If you use a Diskus, remember that once the device is cocked, it must remain in a level position. Exhaling into the device will cause humidity and moistening of the powder inside. The counter indicates the number of doses remaining. Do not take your Diskus apart.

To use your Diskus, perform the following steps:

1. Hold the Diskus flat, rotating it open until it clicks.

2. To expose the dose, rotate the lever until you hear another click.

3. Turn your head to the side and exhale through pursed lips until your lungs feel completely empty.

4. Keeping the device level, put the mouthpiece up to your lips and inhale deep and fast.

5. Hold the powder in your lungs for at least 10 seconds.

6. Relax, and exhale normally away from the device. (Remember, exhaling into the device will create humidity and cause the powder to clump.)

7. Close the Diskus.

8. Check the counter on the side of the Diskus. It should have decreased by one number. Take note of the dosages remaining. When you get to five doses left, the number will appear in red for the remaining doses, alerting you that it is time to refill your prescription.

9. If your Diskus contains a steroidal medication, rinse your mouth completely with water, spitting the water out. (Do not swallow it.)

HOW TO USE A FLEXHALER

If you use a Flexhaler, remember that it must be primed prior to the initial use and for each additional dose thereafter. Keep it in an upright position during this priming. The dose counter on the Flexhaler indicates the number of doses remaining in intervals of tens, and when you see a zero in a red background, it is indication that the Flexhaler is empty. It would be a good idea to track your doses to ensure that you refill your prescription before your device is empty.

To use your Flexhaler, perform the following steps:

1. Hold the device upright, grasping the brown bottom part with one hand and the white lid with the other.
2. Twist gently to remove the white cover.
3. Hold the device by the brown grip, in the upright position, in one hand.
4. Using the thumb and index finger of your other hand, grasp the inhaler in the middle. *Do not hold the inhaler at the top of the mouthpiece.*
5. Twist the brown grip as far as it will go in one direction and then fully back again in the other direction until it stops. It doesn't matter which way you turn it first. You will hear a clicking sound during one of the twisting movements.
6. Repeat step 3.
7. Your inhaler is now primed. Do not shake the inhaler.
8. Turn your head away from inhaler, and exhale until your lungs feel empty.
9. Place inhaler in your mouth, sealing your lips around it.
10. Inhale quick and deeply. You may not sense the presence of any medication, or taste it. This does not mean the dose was not administered. Do not take an additional dose if you do not feel or taste the medication.
11. Hold the powder in your lungs for 10 seconds.
12. Remove the inhaler from your mouth, and turn your head to exhale. (Remember, it is not a good idea to exhale into the device, as it may cause the powder to clump.)
13. Replace the cover onto the device.
14. Rinse your mouth with water, spitting the water out. (Do not swallow.)

HOW TO USE AN ASMANEX TWISTHALER

If you use an Asmanex Twisthaler, the best way to prepare it for use is to simply remove the cap. A dose counter, located at the base of the device, counts down each time the cap is removed. As with any inhaler, it is a good idea to track how many doses you have left. With this inhaler, as soon as it is empty you will no longer be able to remove the top. When the counter reads "01," you will have one dose left. After the administration of that dose, when the cap is returned, you will no longer be able to remove it. At this time, you can throw the device away. Remember, again, to turn your head away from the device upon exhalation. You don't want to put any humidity into the Twisthaler as it can cause the powder to clump up, disrupting the delivery of the medication.

To use your Twisthaler, perform the following steps:

1. Hold the Twisthaler straight up, so the pink base is at the bottom.
2. Twist the white cap counterclockwise.
3. Remove the cap.
4. Breathe out normally, exhaling until your lungs are empty, but turn your head so as to not exhale into the Twisthaler.
5. Place the Twisthaler in your mouth, forming a seal around it with your lips.
6. Inhale quickly and deeply. You may not feel or taste any medication as you inhale. Do not take another dose. When you twisted the cap, it released the powder into place for inhalation. Even though you may not feel or taste the medication, you inhaled it from the device.
7. Remove the device from your mouth.
8. Hold your breath for 10 seconds.
9. Turn your head away from the device and exhale.
10. Wipe the mouthpiece and return the cap to the Twisthaler. Line up the arrow on the cap with the dose counter window, and turn clockwise. When you hear the click, the arrow will line up with the window on the pink base. This will show you how many doses are left in the Twisthaler.
11. If you need another dose, repeat the steps.

Nebulizers

Nebulizers have a few advantages for themselves that make it a perfect fit for some people. The nebulizer is less dependent on patient coordination and cooperation, a breath hold is not required, and the drug concentration can be modified, if necessary.

On the downside, nebulizers can be expensive, bulky, and time-consuming. Correct medication output is device dependent—and not all nebulizers are created equal.

If you are using a nebulizer, a traditional filling volume will be 3 to 5 ml per dose, the airflow to the nebulizer will be close to 6 to 8 L/min, and your average treatment time will be approximately 10 minutes. To use a nebulizer, you simply use your regular breathing pattern, with an occasional deep breath and hold (this will increase medication being deposited into your lungs).

The more you use your nebulizer, the more familiar you will become with it and the greater your comfort level will be. You will realize such things as whether there is a disruption of some sort in the airflow and whether the attachments are correct. You will become familiar with the sputter sound you will hear toward the end of your treatment. You will also gain greater comfort with filling your nebulizer with your medications, cleaning your nebulizer (properly, to prevent infection, check the manufacturer's recommendations and/or the rules for cleaning that follow), and proper assembly of the machine (again, check with your manufacturer's recommendations).

Here are a few things to remember when using a nebulizer:

- Be sure to wash your hands prior to handling the equipment or supplies.
- Clean the equipment as recommended, always start your therapy with clean equipment and parts, and always wash the parts afterward.
- Remember to store your medications properly, and check their expiration dates to ensure you are receiving adequate treatment.

CLEANING YOUR NEBULIZER

After each session or treatment, do the following:

- Tip the cup upside down, and tap or shake any dead volume from the cup.
- Rinse the cup with distilled or sterile water, shake out (do not wipe), and air dry.

To clean the equipment, do the following:

- First, wash your hands to prevent the spread of germs.
- Wash your nebulizer and/or mouthpiece or mask daily in warm, soapy water. Rinse in warm water, shake out, and air dry.
- To disinfect your nebulizer, there are a few options you can use, depending on your manufacturer's recommendations. You may soak the equipment (nonelectrical parts such as tubing and cup only) in the following:
  - Acetic acid (vinegar) for approximately 1 hour
  - A diluted bleach/water solution (1 part bleach to 50 parts water) for approximately 3 minutes
  - Isopropyl alcohol for 5 minutes
  - Boiling in water for 5 minutes
  - Hydrogen peroxide for 30 minutes

Or, in the top rack in your dishwasher, run through a full cycle.

If you use a chemical to clean your equipment, remember to rinse with sterile water afterward, and again, air dry without wiping.

HOW TO USE A RESPIMAT INHALER

There is one last inhaler that doesn't fit neatly into the previous categories. Respimat is a newer "propellant-free" inhaler that uses a slow-moving mist (similar to that from a nebulizer) to deliver its medication.

The Respimat inhaler comes with a dose counter to help you track your dosages. It can be found on the side of the inhaler in the form of a clear plastic strip with a red arrow beneath it. It will point toward different "zones" of green and red and will have numbers in increments of thirty along the side of the color strip. The pointer will move with each dose, and will indicate how much medication you have left. When you reach the red zone, you will have thirty doses left, or seven days of recommended dosing. Once you reach the end of the dosages, the inhaler will automatically lock, preventing further use.

This type of inhaler is different from what you have used in the past. It generates a slow-moving mist for you to inhale. Remember that this is different from a propelled inhaler, and it might feel different to use. If you feel as if you didn't get "enough" medication, remember that it is not safe to take another dose without speaking with your physician or health-care provider. Each Respimat inhaler contains enough puffs, or doses, of medication to last thirty days. Your physician may prescribe you the recommended dosage, or your prescription may be different depending upon what your health-care provider feels is best for you.

For your first use, you will need to install the medication cartridge. With the orange cap closed (I refer here to Combivent brand colors), press the safety cap and pull *off* the clear base. Inside the cap will be a piercing element. Be careful not to touch this. This is used to poke a hole in the bottom of the cartridge to allow for airflow. Next, write the "discard by date" on the inhaler (it will be three months from the date of the prescription).

Once you install the cartridge into the inhaler, it should not be removed. The cartridge will not be flush with the bottom of the container. Once this is inserted, place the clear base back in place. This base will not be removed again during the use of this cartridge.

To prime the inhaler prior to first use, complete these steps:

1. Hold the container upright, keeping the orange cap closed.
2. Turn the base half a turn, or until it "clicks" into place.
3. Open the orange cap so it is fully open.
4. Press "dose release button" while pointing the end of the container away from yourself, toward the floor.
5. Close the orange cap, and repeat these steps until you see the medication mist dispersed from the container.
6. Once you see the mist expelled from the inhaler, repeat these steps another three times to ensure proper priming. (Don't worry, this will not reduce the number of effective dosages delivered from this cartridge. You will still get the full 120 doses.)

7. Your Respimat inhaler is now ready to use.

Now that your inhaler is properly primed and ready to use, let's review the steps necessary for your daily dosing.

1. Hold the inhaler upright, with the orange cap closed to avoid accidental dose release.
2. Turn the base half a turn, or until it "clicks" into place.
3. Open the orange cap fully.
4. Take a breath in, and exhale slowly using pursed lip breathing to expel as much air as you can.
5. Place your lips around the top of the inhaler mouthpiece.
6. Point the inhaler to the back of your throat.
7. While taking in a slow, deep breath, press the dose release button. Inhale as deeply as you can.
8. Hold your breath for 10 seconds.
9. Close the Respimat inhaler cap until it locks into place.

If three days have passed since the last time you used your inhaler, release one dose of medication to properly prime inhaler for use. If it has been twenty-one days, follow the last three steps in the priming instructions to prepare for proper dosage.

To care for your inhaler, clean the inside of the mouthpiece with a dry tissue at least weekly. You can wipe the outside off with a damp cloth. Do not use any of the wet-wash methods described for the other devices. Your inhaler should be stored at room temperature.

FLARE-UPS—AND HOW TO MANAGE THEM

Exacerbation is a medical term for a flare-up, or attack, of your COPD symptoms. Put simply, it means that your symptoms worsen to the point where your regular medications are not sufficient to control them anymore.

Write It Down! My Medications and Refill Calendar

Turn to the chart on page 292 in the Appendix to record ALL the medications you are taking (don't forget over-the-counter meds and supplements), including the name, dosage, frequency, whether it is a rescue medicine or for maintenance, and the doctor who prescribed it. Be sure to note any side effects you experience when taking a particular medication.

Then, photocopy and use the My Monthly Medications: Refill Calendar chart on page 294 of the Appendix for a visual reminder of when you are supposed to refill each medication (or use a blank calendar of your own). After dating it for each appropriate month, mark the day each prescription is filled, calculate the number of days your dosages allow prior to needing a refill, and then mark one week prior to that day to call the pharmacist for a refill, as well as the day you will pick your prescriptions up. Then repeat for each additional month.

You are familiar with your normal. This normal is your baseline. Anything that deviates from your baseline needs to be listened to, and you need to be aware of these changes in your symptoms and condition. Keep in mind that your symptoms may very well change somewhat from day to day—meaning your morning cough may be worse than your afternoon cough, you may have more mucus production in the evening hours than at lunchtime, or vice versa. Your breathing will be easier or more difficult for a few reasons at various times of day. This is not an exacerbation. This is normal. Your symptoms will change during differing times of day. Pay attention to this, and use it to help establish your baseline.

So, if those daily "swings" of symptoms are normal, then what is an exacerbation? What are the specific signs you should watch for? Look at the following list; your exacerbation may include all of these, and it may just include some. It may also include unlisted things that are specific to you. What is important is that you are aware of the changes, as well as how persistent they become. If, at any time, there is a change that worsens your symptoms and persists beyond just a few days, always contact your physician. Some of the changes you may want to watch for, and will likely experience during an exacerbation, are:

- Increased sputum (mucus production) and cough
- Change in the consistency of your mucus (thicker, stickier)
- Change in color (indicates infection)
- Increased wheezing
- Chest tightness
- Fever

Write It Down!
My Exacerbation (Flare-Up) Symptoms

Until you are used to your norm, or if you feel it changing, record your symptoms on the chart on page 300 of the Appendix. This will help you establish and understand what you can expect each day. This will ease your anxiety and decrease your tension, which both greatly affect your ability to breathe your best. You want to remember that an exacerbation varies from these daily swings in that an exacerbation necessitates a change in medication, and sometimes more, to regain control of your symptoms. Note: If you have asthma, see page 157, for more information about asthma exacerbations.

What causes exacerbations? Evidence shows that smoking and air pollution are great factors. Infection is also a primary contributor to the worsening of symptoms. This is why it is essential that you pay attention to your mucus. It can give indication, through coloring and consistency, of what is occurring. Fever is also another indication of infection. Approximately one third of exacerbations occur without either of these factors being present, the very reason that it is important for you to be familiar with your baseline. These exacerbations may be due to various reasons, including possible nonadherence or improper use of medications, inactivity, weather changes, humidity, dry air, excessive cold or heat, and more. Some of the reasons for this occurring are hard to pinpoint because of the variations in individuals and their symptoms.

The good news is that using your medications properly will help you avoid exacerbations. Additionally, keeping up your activity level and participating in an effective pulmonary rehabilitation program (see Step 6) decreases the likelihood of exacerbations by up to 60 percent.

It is important that you record the usage of your medications. You will likely have controller medications that you take every day. These are your maintenance medications. You will take these every day, just as directed. You will also have rescue medications. These will be used when your maintenance medications are not sufficient. This may change a little, day to day, or as mentioned earlier, during different times of the day. What matters most is that you track your normal usage for your rescue medication. Many times, the first indication of an upcoming exacerbation is not a change in your mucus, a different or more persistent or productive cough, or a fever, but simply a persistent need for an increased amount of your rescue medication. If this occurs, notice it. Write it down. Know the number of days and amount of usages you require so you can let your physician know. Again, *make note of anything that deviates from your normal or your baseline.*

Tracking Asthma/COPD Exacerbations

An asthma exacerbation is an attack or an increase of difficulty breathing, wheezing, mucus production, coughing, or decreased pulmonary function. It can be an extremely scary situation. Your asthma/COPD action plan will help you assess the severity of your flare-up and help you track what situations or triggers initiate it. It will also help make you familiar with and feel confident in managing your exacerbations, help you determine what level of treatment your exacerbations require, and help you decide at what point you should call your physician or visit the emergency department, if necessary.

> ### Write It Down! My Asthma Exacerbations and Rescue Medications
>
> Be sure to track your medication administration and your exacerbation record. This will help your physician (as well as you) know the effectiveness of your asthma treatments.
>
> Using the charts on pages 300 and 299 of the Appendix will help outline the effectiveness of your asthma/COPD treatment. Insert the date and time in which your exacerbation took place. Track any missed doses of your controller medication for your record. Write down what allergen or irritant you may have been exposed to prior to your exacerbation. Take this with you to your physician appointments, so your physician can more directly decide whether your asthma is being managed appropriately and effectively.

INFECTION CONTROL

Infection control lies in the palms of your hands, literally. You've heard over and over again that washing your hands is your best line of defense against infection, and it is so true. Every time you go to the store, touch a door knob, or enter any public place, especially during cold and flu season, you place yourself at increased risk of infection. It is important that you take responsibility for the things you can control in regard to it. Practice the following healthy habits to reduce your chance of infection:

- Wash your hands regularly, especially prior to eating, preparing food, or touching your medications. Engage your family and loved ones in a clean-hands campaign for your health and encourage everyone you come in contact with to wash their hands frequently, especially when in contact with you.
- Wear a mask to prevent the inhalation of airborne illness.
- Disinfect doorknobs, light switches, and surface areas in your home with disinfectant wipes regularly.

- Don't visit hospitals, physician offices, or other health-care settings unless it is really necessary.
- Don't visit or have visitors come to you that are ill or feverish.
- Maintain a healthy diet, including vitamins and minerals to boost your immune system.
- Maintain a healthy lifestyle, including exercise and staying active to boost your immune system.
- Reduce stress and practice relaxation techniques to boost your immune system.

HAVING AN ASTHMA OR COPD ACTION PLAN

An action plan is a guide you can use to monitor the control of your asthma or COPD symptoms. You will see, by reading through the action plans (see pages 296–297 in the Appendix), that they are a great way to track the effectiveness of your medications in treating your asthma or COPD. The green, yellow, and red zones list symptoms of asthma and COPD. As each person is unique, these lists do not attempt to be comprehensive; thus, some of your symptoms may be different. The actions column lists recommendations for you or your health-care provider to take based upon your symptoms, and your provider may write down other actions that are unique to your needs. Using an action plan can help you better control your asthma or COPD. It's been shown to reduce emergency department visits, work absences, nighttime flare-ups, and hospitalizations in those who use it.

Using Your Asthma/COPD Action Plan

Review your asthma/COPD action plan. Get familiar with it and comfortable with each section. You can assign your own personal numbers to each percentage that is listed. For example, if your daily average peak flow measurement is 360, that value would fall into the green zone for

Write It Down!
My Asthma/COPD Action Plan

Fill in the action plans (see pages 296 and 297 of the Appendix) that apply to you, so that you will have a set of symptoms and instructions for whenever you have a flare-up.

you. The same goes for symptom management. You know what symptoms are normal for you on a daily basis, and those fall into the green zone. After determining what your normal is, you will be able to assign a zone in your action plan for each numeric value or symptom you have. This will be useful as you monitor your daily peak flow values and watch for any change in your symptoms. When you begin to see a decrease in your peak flow values, an increase in mucus production or cough, fever, difficulty breathing, or other symptom changes that alter from your normal it could mean there is a change in your zone. Knowing this, you will be able to manage your flare-up under the guidelines given in your action plan.

Now let's look at the zones listed in your action plan. You can see that a healthy zone—the green zone—is where you want to be. The yellow zone is a warning zone used to serve as a guideline to treating your symptoms. When you find yourself in this zone, you will need to have your rescue breather. You will take two to six puffs of your rescue breather every 20 minutes, followed by a repeat of your peak flow. Be sure to record your results so you can monitor them for either an improvement or a decrease in your symptoms. Repeat this for one hour, at which time you will need to evaluate your position.

- Have you improved? If so, continue to take your rescue breather once every hour, monitoring your peak flows after each dose.
- Have you worsened? If you have worsened, contact your physician. **The red zone in your action plan requires emergency help.** If you, at any time, you find yourself in the red zone (signs would be losing color in your face or fingers, and blue/purple- or gray-tinged lips, nose, or fingernails), call an ambulance and get to the nearest hospital emergency

department immediately. Have a loved one take the written records you have made, including your asthma action plan, with you to the hospital.

As you can see, using this plan, taking your medications regularly and as prescribed, knowing the proper way to take your medications, and tracking your condition daily is the only effective way to manage your disease.

> ## Asthma Tracker Reminder
>
> - **Green zone:** 80 to 100 percent of your personal best; symptoms well controlled
> - **Yellow zone:** 50 to 79 percent of your personal best. Use a rescue breather (quick relief) and other medications as directed to improve symptoms.
> - **Red zone:** Less than 50 percent of your personal best. Increase your rescue breather and call your physician or go to the emergency room.

When an asthma emergency takes place, there is little time for anything but directly managing your symptoms. When you can't breathe, nothing else really matters. Part of successfully managing this disease also includes keeping track of your medication dosages. Some of your inhalers will have counters on them to track the doses; some of them will not.

MEASURING PEAK FLOW

Using a peak flow meter is a good way to track the symptoms you are experiencing, as well as alert yourself and your health-care providers to any changes that may lead to an exacerbation. If you do not have a peak flow meter, you may ask your physician to prescribe you one.

Peak flow meter readings should be taken upon waking, during your best time of day, and after the use of your quick relief (rescue) medications. The optimal time of day to do it is first thing in the morning, prior to using your medications. However, it is a good idea to find a time of day that works best for you. You need to repeat the measurements at the same time every day. You also need to use the same meter, and when replacing it, use the same brand of meter to ensure the readings

Write It Down! My Monthly Dose Counter

To know approximately how long your inhaler will last, determine how many dosages or actuations your inhaler has. Next, calculate approximately how many doses you use daily, and divide the original amount of actuation by the amount of "puffs" you use each day. This will tell you how many days your medication will last. Make note of this in the chart on page 295 of the Appendix, write the refill date in permanent marker on your inhaler, and call for a refill of your prescription one week before the estimated date of last available dose. This will provide you with constant medication.

will be most accurate and enable you to have a truer tracking of your symptoms.

For instance, after you take your peak flow upon waking, perhaps ten or eleven a.m. is your best time of day. Measure your peak flow and record it at that time each day, as well as, say, after your three p.m. bronchodilator. Doing this will help you determine which zone you are in when recorded and used as part of your asthma action plan, which can direct you to the correct care for your symptoms. Your medications should enable you to remain in the green zone without using your rescue breather more than twice per week. If you use your rescue breather more frequently than that, you may need to have your controller medication adjusted.

To measure your peak flow, follow these directions:

1. Move the indicator to the bottom of the numbered scale.
2. Stand up.
3. Exhale through pursed lips, emptying your lungs completely.
4. Inhale, filling your lungs completely.
5. Place the mouthpiece of the peak flow meter in your mouth.
6. Exhale into it as hard and as fast as you can (in a single blow).
7. Record your reading.

8. Repeat these steps two more times, and record your best (highest) reading in your tracker sheet.

WHEN EXACERBATIONS ARE SEVERE

Sometimes exacerbations require a hospital stay. This, of course, is something everybody wants to avoid. So, it's important to be aware of what your symptoms are and how they have changed. By doing this, and taking this information to your physician in the early stages of your exacerbation, you may be able to avoid a hospitalization or emergency room visit. Taking charge and being aggressive in treating the flare-ups may help decrease their duration and severity.

> **Write It Down! My Peak Expiratory Flow (PEF) Tracking Sheet**
>
> Use the chart on page 295 in the Appendix to keep track of your peak flows.

Finding yourself hospitalized with an exacerbation can be overwhelming and frightening. If this happens, please try to let yourself relax, as stress and anxiety oftentimes can increase your difficulties. Following your health-care practitioners' instructions and working with them to adjust your medications to gain control of your symptoms will be one of the best things you can do for yourself.

In severe cases, you may find yourself in respiratory failure, requiring a ventilator for support. Let's review a few things about this situation, for your understanding.

Ventilators

Ventilators are used to support those who, for various reasons, cannot maintain a respiratory effort sufficient to support themselves on their own. There are various types of ventilators, but all have the same goal: to support the patient in the best possible way.

What About Advance Directives and Resuscitation?

Advance directives and resuscitation are difficult topics, ones that you know should be addressed but may not want to because it's scary for you and for your family. But it's very important to be clear on these issues—it can make a tremendous difference in the long run.

Resuscitation is a word used in situations where the patient is unconscious and/or nearing death. The primary efforts to keep you alive are usually made by trained professionals and are usually followed by transportation to a hospital to continue and extend such lifesaving measures.

With some advance planning, you can be sure you will have a voice in such matters: You may choose to enact a living will or a "do not resuscitate" (DNR) order in cases where you do not want lifesaving measures to be taken for you or on your behalf. A living will or DNR as well as durable power of attorney are legal documents that are put into place to respect your wishes. They outline what you prefer to have happens in situations or under circumstances in which you would not be able to communicate or make the required decision, such as if you were unconscious, in a coma, or in other emergency situations. The decisions to put any of these documents into action are typically made in advance of crisis by a person for him- or herself, are sometimes based upon illness or age, and are based completely upon the individual's personal choices. If a DNR or living will is not in place stating specifically that you prefer otherwise, lifesaving measures will be taken in emergency and other situations.

Another option you may want to think about is having a health-care proxy. A health-care proxy is someone—a family member or friend you are close to—who is authorized to make health-care decisions for you if you lose the ability to make decisions for yourself. This "health-care agent" can make sure that the health-care providers responsible for you are following your wishes regarding your health and care. He or she can also make decisions if your medical condition changes, and make your physicians aware of your plans. You can choose how much authority you wish to give your health-care proxy, allowing him or her to make all the decisions that need to be made, or only a few. You may also give your proxy specific instructions that he or she has to follow in regard to your care. Your attorney can help you follow all guidelines for your state or area of residence to ensure that your wishes are heeded.

It isn't fun to think about, but nevertheless it is important to evaluate now what you would like to have happen in the event of a difficult situation. Ask yourself, "How many heroic efforts do I want made on my behalf?" and "Do I want my life to be sustained, and if so, for how long?" If you do not want lifesaving measures to be taken, or you would like them to be limited to specific circumstances, it is important that you put your requests in writing so your desires are clear to everyone involved. Establishing these desires in a legal document will ease the burden on your family, friends, loved ones, and health-care providers in situations where you will not be able to state what you want for yourself. As they may be faced with some very difficult decisions under these circumstances, it will ease the decision-making process for them and offer them the reassurance that your wants and desires are being respected and met.

If this is something you would like to do, plan ahead by talking to your health-care provider or an attorney to establish the parameters you would like to set for yourself, and to appoint a durable power of attorney (who need not be an actual attorney). Take control of this situation, and ease your anxiety by making your desires known to those that matter.

What Is Hospice?

Hospice is a service that is used to ease the burden of patients and their loved ones during the last stages of life. It is a type of care that is based upon the philosophy of focusing on relieving and preventing suffering of the terminally ill patient. Hospice addresses issues such as physical, emotional, spiritual, or social difficulties in hope of making the transition through each stage of end of life as comfortable as possible for all involved.

Keep in mind that while it is designed for end-of-life care, that "end-of life" does not always mean days or hours. It can last for months, if necessary. Hospice is a service that typically streamlines all the patient medications, nursing, and other clinical care through a specific agency, allowing for a greater awareness of each particular situation, family, and patient to be available to all the caretakers. This can be invaluable to the family members of the patient because it may ease the weight of caring for their loved one, enabling them to focus more heavily upon coping with their own emotions as the physical needs of the loved one are met through appropriate providers. Some agencies provide help to the extent of housekeeping and clergy to complete the degree of assistance the family can receive.

Again, while it may not be the most pleasant thing to think about, at some point in time, many may reach a stage that will qualify them for hospice. Some people find the notion and philosophy of hospice a comfort; others may not find it useful and may not be attracted to it, or may have a large enough family surrounding them that it is not necessary or desired. Either way, focusing on the comfort of the patient needs to be the primary concern of everyone involved.

Whatever situation you may be in, talk to your loved ones about the possibility of hospice as a help when the time comes and decide if it is for you. Your physician can direct you to the correct agencies in your area if it is something that you feel you would like to pursue at any time.

Some ventilators require a tube (called an endotracheal tube, or ET) to be inserted into your lungs to provide you with the air necessary to breathe. Other types use a mask that covers your mouth and nose, or in some cases your entire face, to provide you with the necessary air to help you breathe. Oxygen is then usually entrained (directed) into the circuit (the tubing the air goes through) leading from the ventilator to either your mask or your ET.

The ventilator will be set according to what your expected lung capacity is or to a pressure that your lungs will tolerate in a positive way. Your lung capacity will be determined by your height and expected lung size. Once this is determined, the machine will be set and will breathe for you until you are capable of doing so on your own.

While you are on the ventilator, you will be monitored, and your settings will be checked frequently to ensure that it is working optimally for you. Your breathing medications can be given to you through your circuit. When you are ready to have the tube taken out, tests will be done to ensure that you are capable of breathing on your own. When the tube is removed, you will likely sit up in your bed and be talked through the procedure. After the tube is removed, you will most likely be put on oxygen (probably an oxygen mask at first) to maintain healthy oxygen saturation levels. You may be given some inhaled medication to help ease you back into breathing on your own, if necessary.

Once you are stable and breathing on our own, the oxygen mask will be converted to a nasal cannula (which you may already be used to) and things will begin to feel more normal. Upon discharge from the hospital, you may have new and/or different medications or dosages. You may also have been prescribed a different liter flow for your oxygen. Keep in mind that this possibly higher liter flow of oxygen may be a temporary thing; don't panic over it. You are establishing a new normal, once again, and your energy would be best used allowing your body to recover rather than worrying about what the new changes are. Give yourself some time to get used to these changes, and to recover. Allow yourself time to heal, and provide your body with the energy it needs to heal by resting and getting the best nutrition you can. Follow your physician's orders, keep your follow-up visits, and take your new medications as directed. Try to be patient with yourself, and allow yourself the right to rest. This, too, shall pass.

Combining the advice in Steps 1 through 5 of this program is the best way for this program to work. It is similar to what you should receive from a strong, effective pulmonary rehab program that is well rounded, includes all necessary elements, and that teaches and helps you implement lifestyle modifications to allow you to continue with your life in a way that makes you happy. But what would those include? The next chapter will give you all the details.

Go to Pulmonary Rehab

When I loved myself enough, I began leaving whatever wasn't healthy. This meant people, jobs, my own beliefs, and habits—anything that kept me small. My judgment called it disloyal. Now I see it as self loving.

—KIM MCMILLEN

To support your circle of therapies to help slow the progression of your lung disease, improve your daily life, and decrease your symptoms, ask your doctor for a referral to a pulmonary rehab (PR) program. Without question, *pulmonary rehab should be part of your pulmonary therapy.* PR is a program designed to help improve your physical, emotional, and psychological health. It includes education about relaxation, breathing techniques, medication adherence, and creating the ability for you to safely establish limits and recovery. Over the course of your treatment, PR will help you better understand the how's and why's of lung disease, recommend adjustments you can make to improve your lifestyle, and suggest ways to make it easier for you to perform your daily obligations.

If you have recently been diagnosed with lung disease, you may feel anxious about the changes in store for you or worried about your future and those you love. These feelings are all normal, and attending a pulmonary rehab program can help you deal with those emotions.

Your goals for PR should include the following:

- Help control respiratory infections
- Increase your physical abilities
- Improve ventilation and cardiac status and ability
- Manage airways and retrain breathing
- Receive medication education
- Find patient and family education and support
- Reduce hospitalizations and medical costs

Write It Down! My Rehab Goals

Take a moment to consider what some of your rehab goals are. Write them down in your journal. Now, think about your concerns. Be honest and write them in your journal, too.

PULMONARY REHAB: THE KEY TO THE COPD SOLUTION

PR is a therapy with well-documented benefits and results for the treatment of patients with debilitating chronic obstructive pulmonary disease (COPD) and other lung diseases. It is considered a standard of care for patients suffering from these conditions. Over the past few decades, there have been several documents published about its effectiveness, but surprisingly, not much has been said of its roots. Let's review the path that guided PR into the product it is today, and how a program will benefit you.

Common knowledge to anybody who either has the disease or loves someone who does is that the major debilitating symptom of COPD is dyspnea, or shortness of breath (SOB), especially with activity. Because of the hindrance this symptom places upon its sufferer, for many years patients were told by their physicians to not exert themselves to the point of losing their breath. They were advised to avoid activities that led to SOB. But following this advice put patients in what is called the anxiety/dyspnea deconditioning cycle, which I call the COPD Downward Spiral:

Not exerting themselves to the point of dyspnea would lead patients into a vicious cycle of not moving around, losing their muscle tone, weakening them, and leading them further and further into disability.

In the 1950s, a contrary opinion was offered for the treatment of this disease. Alvan L. Barach, MD, Columbia University–New York, was a pioneer in pulmonary medicine. His studies revealed that not only did oxygen therapy offer much needed relief and assistance to his pulmonary patients but also that those who *exercised* with oxygen showed considerable improvement in their capacity to exercise without oxygen. In other words, they showed an improved ability to perform activities (such as walking) without feeling short of breath. Dr. Barach saw a positive physiological response in his patients. He learned that exercise, even for breathless people, is one of the ways by which they can restore physical fitness.

Another pulmonologist, considered to be of the most accomplished of his generation, was Thomas L. Petty, MD. Affiliated with the University of Colorado, Dr. Petty and his group have been credited with the official organization of the standardized outpatient pulmonary rehabilitation program. His program offered his patients the following:

- Individualized instruction about the disease
- Information about bronchial hygiene
- Breathing retraining techniques
- Physical reconditioning
- Individualized drug therapy

Through his work, exercise conditioning was defined as an essential component to the treatment of COPD.

Shown to improve shortness of breath, increase exercise tolerance, and increase quality of life to a *greater* degree than *any other single COPD therapy used today,* pulmonary rehab has proven effective over decades of study and debate. Your physician knows this, which is why he or she may prescribe this therapy for you. Where do you go from there?

By reading this book, you're already on your way to a PR plan that will work for you. First, let's look at the anxiety/dyspnea deconditioning cycle.

THE ANXIETY/DYSPNEA DECONDITIONING CYCLE

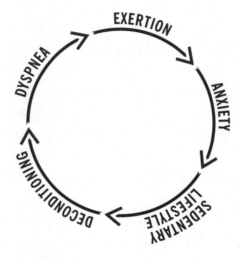

As you can see from the diagram, falling into a cycle of deconditioning is easy to do, and can sometimes be difficult to escape. It is common to become alarmed when activities become difficult to perform. It is also common to have high levels of anxiety if you have difficulty breathing. The good news is, this cycle can be stopped and turned around. You *can* succeed. You *can* improve. You can find yourself in a better place with more enjoyment and a greater ability to live.

Some tissues in your body can regenerate after an accident or illness. If you break a bone or cut your skin, your body kicks into hyperdrive, dispatching all the appropriate, designated "armed forces" to the area of damage to repair what is broken and make you whole again. Unfortunately, lung tissue doesn't fall under the "armed forces" umbrella. The tissue cannot be regenerated. This means that once the damage is done, it cannot be undone.

So, if your lung tissue cannot be repaired, how does PR help? What you are changing with this therapy is the degree of efficiency of oxygen consumption at the cellular level. In other words, you are making your muscles more efficient. You are training them to work better with less oxygen. When this happens, more oxygen remains available in your blood. When there is more available oxygen, more of your tissues receive it, and you, in turn, feel fewer episodes of SOB. The cycle reverses! This is why it is important for you to remain persistent in your therapy.

What this means, in reference to PR, is that you are going to work to improve your ability to actively participate in your day-to-day life, to move and do the things that need to be done each day, as well as those things you simply find enjoyable. As PR is an exercise-based program, with many other elements combined to complete it, you can expect to work. You can also expect to see results in your ability to perform. You will see increased strength, decreased SOB, increased endurance, and increased anxiety management. You'll get a good understanding of nutrition and how it affects your body. Most of all, you will find that you feel better—all over.

Your therapist will watch your vital signs during your visit. Your therapist will keep you safe. Your focus should be on lifting 2 more pounds or performing two more repetitions. Your focus should be on strengthening those muscles and walking that extra 100 feet. Your focus should be on using relaxation techniques and envisioning in your mind your success. Your focus should be on your breathing exercises. You will see success. It happens every single day.

WHAT WILL YOUR PR THERAPY CONSIST OF?

Your therapy will involve a multidisciplinary approach to treat you as a whole, instead of addressing only individual symptoms. Here are some of the things a typical PR program consists of. You'll recognize that many of these things are included in the COPD Solution program in this book, which is based on PR. Attending a PR program and meeting with therapists on a regular basis will help you meet your goals—and support you every step of the way.

Physical reconditioning: You will begin your exercise routine at a level determined by your own tolerance. It will be decided on during your PR evaluation. Your program will be designed specifically for you, with your limitations taken into consideration. Your therapist's goal will be to improve your physical health while maintaining your oxygen saturation levels. You will be involved in both cardio and strength training. Well-conditioned muscles require less energy and offer more efficient oxygen consumption. And remember, exercise *can* be fun. You will learn ways to incorporate exercises you will enjoy into your life and enhance your lifestyle (we'll talk about exercise on pages 175–177).

Emotional reconditioning: Sometimes disease can bring about big changes in our lives that can overwhelm us and be difficult to deal with. You will be evaluated to see what level your emotions are presently at. If you meet the requirements and would like to meet with a counselor, an appointment will be set up for you to do so. For more on this, see Step 1, page 73.

Breathing retraining: The way you have spent your entire life breathing may not work for you anymore. Did you know there are things that can make breathing easier and more effective? Your therapist will show you exercises to retrain yourself how to breathe, allowing you to get more out of each breath. You can practice these breathing techniques with the recommendations on pages 103–106 in Step 3.

Nutrition: Believe it or not, some of the foods you eat may actually be making it more difficult for you to breathe. For this reason, your therapist will discuss not only healthy eating habits but also foods to avoid that can hinder your ability to perform tasks and maintain the quality of life you would like (and you'll find more information about nutrition in Step 8).

Medications: You will review the different types of medications available to patients with diseases such as yours, ensure you know how and when to use yours correctly, and work with your therapist on answering any questions you may have regarding your medications. Using your medication appropriately is an important part of your therapy (see Step 5, page 129, for more about this).

Infection control: You will discuss the appropriate measures to take to reduce the spread of infection and keep you out of the hospital. See Step 5, page 158.

Smoking cessation: Although many patients have lung disease because they have been smokers, many still continue to smoke. If this applies to you, you will learn the nature of addiction and how you can work with your therapist to overcome it. Step 7 offers some tips for quitting for good.

> Remember . . . this is your body; this is your health. THERE ARE NO DUMB QUESTIONS!

Setting goals: Setting reasonable goals and expectations for yourself will be easier than you think. Once you get started and become familiar with your body and what you are capable of doing, you will help determine what your short- and long-term goals are. As you progress through your program, you will enjoy seeing your progress and feeling the benefits of your success.

Education: You will receive education about any and all aspects of your disease and related problems. Questions and unanswered concerns give cause for fear. Fear gives cause for anxiety. Anxiety makes it harder for you to breathe. Ask questions!

PULMONARY REHAB EXERCISES

The best exercises for the heart, lungs, and circulatory system are called **isotonic** (aerobic) activities, which involve continuous rhythmic

Write It Down!
My Pulmonary Rehab Team

Turn to the chart on page 288 in the Appendix to write down the names of all your PR therapists. A PR team commonly includes a respiratory therapist, physical therapist, occupational therapist, dietitian, and a social worker or counselor.

motion. These include such things as walking, cycling, running, and swimming. Isotonic activities help increase the body's muscle tone, cardiovascular endurance, and strength. For you, that means these exercises will make the largest impact on your ability to move around without feeling short of breath.

Exercises that involve contracting muscle without body movement strengthen specific muscle groups. This is called **isometric** activity. These include lifting, pushing, pulling, and carrying. Isometric activities are beneficial in keeping muscles toned and strengthened but have no real benefit to your cardiovascular system. For you, that means they are important because they will give you extra strength for lifting or moving objects, such as dishes, and other similar activities during your day, but they will not make as much of a difference in your breathing as the isotonic, or aerobic, activities will. It is important for you to incorporate both types of exercise into your routine.

While establishing your exercise routine, consider how hard you should work, or your level of **exertion**. One purpose of exercise is to increase your ability to perform more overtime, or build your endurance and strength as you go. For some, it is hard to determine how hard to work. One way to gauge how hard you should work is to focus on being able to talk while you exercise. You should feel as if you can talk, but maybe don't necessarily want to.

The trouble is that with lung patients, talking during exertion lowers oxygen saturation levels. This creates a problem, as you need as much oxygen as you can get, especially when you are working. For this purpose, do not talk during your exercise, but put yourself in a position in

> ### *Write It Down!*
> ### *My Pulmonary Rehab Schedule*
>
> Using the blank calendar grid on page 288 in the Appendix or a blank calendar of your own (or dedicate a special color of ink for PR in your regular calendar or datebook), mark the days and time you attend therapy. An example would be Monday, Wednesday, and Friday mornings at 10 a.m. Let's assume that on Tuesday, Thursday, and Saturday mornings, you complete some sort of exercise on your own at home. On the days when you exercise at home, note down what exercises you will do there. Be sure to include in your calendar your attendance of any additional classes your therapist offers.

which you feel as if you could. Remember to perform your pursed lip breathing during difficult times. It is okay to stop and rest to do this. Exercise does not have to be strenuous for your body to benefit.

Remember to start each session slowly and warm up. Then cool down. Exercise four to five times per week, starting at the same length of time you did upon your rehab completion. Rest between activities, giving yourself time to recover before moving on to the next activity. Remember to take into consideration weather conditions and your individual triggers, or what sets off your breathing difficulties, when you are establishing your exercise routine, as well. It will not be beneficial to you to be outside walking if the air is full of allergens that cause more difficulty for you. Your exercise routine will and should vary not only to adjust to your needs but also to keep your interest.

WHEN THE GOING GETS TOUGH . . . KEEP GOING!

No one ever said PR is easy. There will be days you want to stop. There will be days you hate your therapist. There will be days you feel as if nothing is helping. There will still be good and bad days. But there will also be days you don't want to stop. There will also be days you love your therapist and what he or she has helped you accomplish. There will also be days you feel as if you have conquered the world.

TAKING PULMONARY REHAB HOME

You may get to the point with your PR that you are capable of continuing this new lifestyle on your own. That is what everybody is hoping for!

First of all, you should congratulate yourself on your accomplishment. If you have reached this point, you have made many changes in your life and have improved your abilities by leaps and bounds. Congratulations on your progress!

Your therapist should have helped you establish a home exercise program (HEP). Your HEP should consist of activities that require no less energy to perform than those you were performing during the final portion of your rehab. You want to continue to progress in your physical fitness, and reducing the amount of activity you do or cutting back a little here and there will take its toll on your body. (Remember how nasty it is to try to play catch-up.) Muscles are like naughty children: They behave badly when not tended to regularly. You will quickly lose muscle tone and endurance if you do not continue on with your activity from the level you are currently at.

Many things can influence your exercise: personal likes and dislikes, access to equipment, seasons (if you live in a seasonal area), and changes in your health. It is important to keep in touch with your physician and keep him or her up to date on your condition, progress, and personal choices.

EASY AT-HOME EXERCISES

It can be really hard to start with exercise, especially if you haven't been moving very much. The good news is that exercise really will help you breathe better. The more strength you build the more efficient your oxygen absorption will be and the better you will be able to perform all your regular activities. When it gets tough, don't give up, keep working at it. Remember to take it step by step and incrementally increase only as you can tolerate it. This will help you continue on, as consistency is the key to these improvements.

Tips: Practice your pursed lip breathing, exhaling through pursed lips as you work the muscle, then inhaling as the muscle group you are working rests. For example, when you lift your leg up, exhale against pursed lips, when you drop it, inhale for fresh oxygen. Most exercises can be performed from a standing and/or sitting position.

Start on your left side and then repeat the exercise on your right side. You can use small hand and ankle weights of 2–3 pounds, if desired, to increase intensity and strength. Repeat ten times for two sets. Perform exercises at home 3–5 days per week.

FRONTAL RAISES

Standing or sitting with back straight and shoulders squared over hips, with your palm facing back, raise arm slowly in front of you to shoulder height and lower it to your side and repeat.

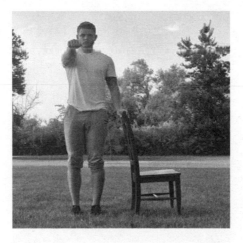

LATERAL RAISES

Standing or sitting with back straight and shoulders squared over hips, with your palm facing inward raise arm slowly at your side to shoulder height and lower it back against your side and repeat.

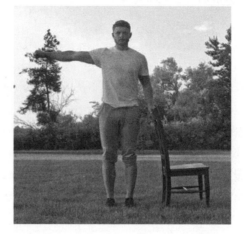

BICEP CURL

With arm hanging at your side, turn hand so palm is facing forward. Raise hand, bending arm at elbow, until it reaches full inward position. Return arm to straightened position at your side and repeat.

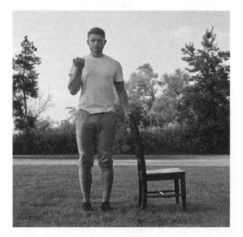

OVERHEAD EXTENSIONS

Take arm from upper bicep curl position with hand facing toward your center and lift arm to straightened position over head. Return to upper curl position and repeat.

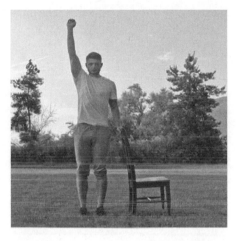

PUSH DOWNS

Hold arm to side with elbow slightly backward and arm bent at a 90 degree angle at the elbow, palm facing inward. Extend arm to straightened position and return to bent position focusing on tightening triceps (muscle in back of arm). Repeat.

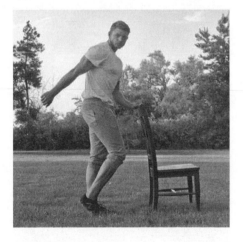

FRONT LEG LIFT

Standing straight with feet shoulder width apart and holding on to the back of a kitchen chair or wall bar for stabilization, lift left leg directly in front of you, toes up, to a 45 degree angle from the ground, then move back to starting position on the ground and repeat.

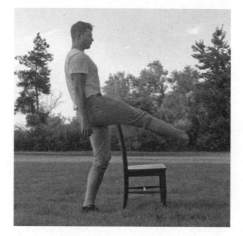

SIDE LEG LIFT

Standing straight with feet shoulder width apart and holding on to the back of a kitchen chair or wall bar for stabilization, lift leg to side keeping foot in neutral position, to a 45 degree angle from the ground, then move back to starting position on the ground and repeat.

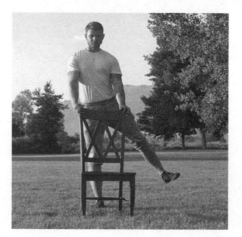

BACK LEG LIFT

Standing straight with feet shoulder width apart and holding on to the back or a kitchen chair or wall bar to stabilize yourself, lift leg backward as far as you can without moving your hips to compensate for the movement, then move your leg back to starting position on the ground and repeat.

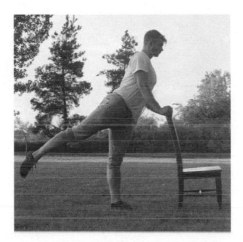

CALF RAISES

Holding on to kitchen chair for stabilization, place feet shoulder width apart and keep feet flat, raise on to toes, then return to starting flat-footed position and repeat.

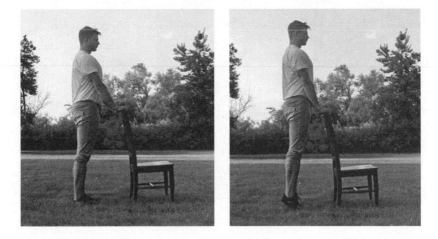

KNEE LIFT

Standing straight with feet shoulder width apart and holding on to the back of a kitchen chair or wall bar for stabilization, bend knee and lift leg to a marching position, then return leg to starting position and repeat.

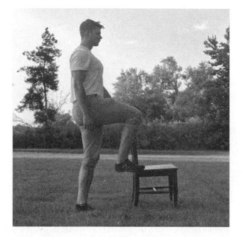

SIT TO STAND

Begin seated on a hard surface, stable chair, then stand up to a full standing position, then return to a seated position, repeat.

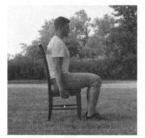 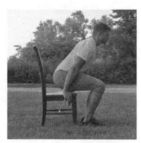 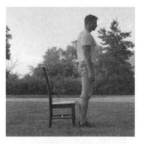

SQUAT

Holding onto the back of a kitchen chair or wall bar for stabilization stand with feet shoulder width apart. Bend at the knee until you are in a seated position and return to standing keeping feet well planted on ground and focusing on placing your weight on the back half of your feet. Repeat.

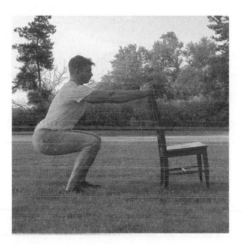

BALANCE STANCE

Begin practicing your balance by standing holding on to the back of a kitchen chair or wall bar for stabilization, lifting one foot off the ground and holding it for a count of thirty, then repeat on the other side. As your balance improves you may advance to having the ability to stand on one foot without stabilizing yourself and holding your arms out to your side for assistance.

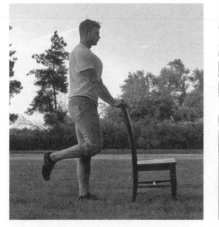 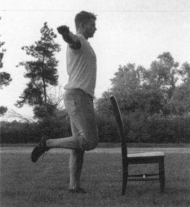

A WORD ABOUT SMOKING AND PR

Sometimes I come across a patient who continues to smoke. If you are still smoking, please keep in mind that the best thing you can do right now is quit. Not only for your own health and that of your family, but for the success of others in your PR program. In fact, there is some debate about whether current smokers should be allowed to participate in pulmonary rehab programs; some programs may not accept clients who smoke, primarily due to concern for the well-being of all participants. If you are a smoker, you may not be aware of how difficult it can be for some of the ex-smokers in rehab to smell the smoke that lingers on your clothing and in your hair while you're in the facility. And even if they have never smoked, some people have a very low tolerance for the odor and their lungs become very irritated when they inhale it, while the smell can make others sick to their stomach. For these reasons, as well as your very own personal ones, participation in a good pulmonary rehab program includes smoking cessation counseling and classes for all who need and want it. The next step focuses on quitting.

Quit Smoking

What you do makes a difference, and you have to decide what kind of difference you want to make.

—JANE GOODALL

You've heard it a thousand times. You need to quit smoking. You may have tried a thousand times. Try one more. You will hear these words again and again:

It is the number one best thing you can do for yourself right now!

And it is. I can't say that enough. Don't let what you may view as past failures keep you from trying again. Quitting is hard, harder for some than others. Smoking may be a habit you have had for ten years, thirty years, or more. But you need to remember these very important things:

You are stronger than your habits.

You are stronger than your cravings.

You are stronger than your past.

Whether your vice is cigarettes or something else, treating the addiction and establishing new routines is of upmost importance. It is more difficult for some than it is for others to quit. For one person, it may take longer, involve a more gradual step down, or require nicotine patches and medications, whereas another person may just wake up one day and call it quits. The key is to not compare yourself to others. That isn't important. What *is* important is that you do what you can, when you can, and that you do a little more just for today. You've heard stories from those that have quit, but here are a few from people in my classes:

> "Quitting was the hardest and best thing I've ever done for myself. There were times I didn't think I could do it, and times I slipped up, but it is all part of the process. If you have a little less today than you did yesterday, you won."

> "For me it was a matter of understanding addiction and knowing it took more than willpower. It's about lifestyle changes. I did it for my grandkids, my son, my wife, and my future. I don't smell like smoke anymore. I can walk farther and do more. It was a great change for me."

> "Quitting, for me, was easy once I decided to do it."

> "I did it for my family, I did it for my friends, I did it for myself. It was hard, but I did it."

If you're thinking about quitting smoking, know that your pulmonary rehabilitation program coordinator understands how difficult it can be. Your PR program should have supportive personnel and resources to help you work with your physician, if necessary, to make this transition into a healthier lifestyle for yourself and your family. If you cannot find resources through your PR program, contact your physician directly. He or she will have medication and contact information for groups and/or therapies available in your area to help you retrain yourself and overcome this roadblock to breathing easier.

Stand right now and give yourself a hand for contemplating this drastic, most healthful change in your life. You deserve it.

REASONS TO QUIT

Quitting smoking can be a difficult thing. This is no secret. It is more difficult for some than others, so be sure not to compare yourself and your efforts to those of others you know, even if they have gone through the same thing. It is important to remember that even if you have quit a hundred times before, you can quit one more time. With the right help and your best effort, YOU CAN DO IT!

Truly, it is the most important thing you can do for yourself right now. Let's review some of the long-term benefits:

- Breathe easier
- Have a healthier heart
- Smell "fresher"
- Reduce your risk of cancer
- Save money
- Have healthier lungs
- Make life healthier for those around you
- Exercise with greater ease

In case you need to give yourself more motivation, take a look at this chart and what happens when you do quit. The benefits kick in immediately! You start breathing easier within minutes and hours. So, with each day that goes by since you've had a cigarette, remember—*you are getting better.*

Talk to your doctor and your respiratory therapist about quitting. They can tell you more about medications and different methods of quitting. Nicotine replacement therapies are popular. Discovering what your triggers are and replacing those with new activities you enjoy will also help you. See the Supportive Online Resources section on page 309 for a list of websites that can help in your efforts to quit.

OKAY, YOU WANT TO QUIT. BUT HOW DO YOU DO IT?

You may not realize it, but you have already started the process of quitting. Just by thinking that you want to quit, in forming that desire in your mind, your journey to being smoke-free has already begun.

What you will do next is dependent on you. You need to pause. You need to think. You need to dwell on giving up cigarettes and review

Stop Smoking Chart

TIME SINCE LAST CIGARETTE	IMPROVEMENT
20 minutes	Increased circulation in hands and feet. Carbon monoxide in cigarettes inhibits the body's ability to carry oxygen.
8 hours	CO_2 levels in blood have returned to normal and blood oxygen levels have returned to normal.
24 hours	Significant decrease in chances of heart attack
48 hours	Your nerve endings will begin to regrow, giving you enhanced smell and taste.
2 weeks	Your circulation will begin improving, and your ability to walk will improve with it.
30 days	You will not be wheezing and coughing as much because the phlegm you cough up will be reduced.
3 months	You will feel a drastic decrease in your shortness of breath, and the sinus problems you may have suffered from will have improved. Your cilia (tiny hairs that move mucus inside your lungs) will return to normal function and will be able to do their job of moving junk out of your lungs. This is going to decrease the number of lung infections you suffer from and improve your lung function!
1 year	Your chances of having heart disease and a heart attack are cut in half. In another four years, your chances of having a stroke returns to that of a nonsmoker.
10 years	Although it will always be higher than a nonsmoker, your chances of having lung cancer have dropped. Also, your risk of getting mouth, throat, esophageal, bladder, kidney, or pancreatic cancer drops. Another 15 years from now, your chances of having coronary artery disease and a heart attack are that of someone who has never smoked.
25 years	Your chances of having coronary artery disease and a heart attack are that of someone who has never smoked.

it again and again in your mind. Part of the process is to focus your energy upon quitting while you are still smoking. Quitting starts long before your last cigarette.

Spend some time evaluating yourself and your habit. Run a typical day through your mind. Break it down, and then write it down. You are going to start with your triggers.

The mind is a funny thing. It is not fixed; it can be trained. Much like Pavlov's dog, who became conditioned to expect food at the sound of a bell, saliva building in his mouth in anticipation of what tasty treats would be placed before him, we often condition ourselves to expect certain things at certain times of the day, in certain places, and under certain circumstances. These are your triggers: the things, places, people, emotions, and circumstances that make you crave a cigarette.

Your next step in quitting is figuring out what your triggers are. Examine your behavior and what feelings or events led up to you needing a smoke break. Write them down. Look at them. Think about them. These are the things you are going to have to avoid and replace after you have your last cigarette. These are the things that are going to make you have to fight to win this war. These are the things that are going to make you stronger and make you search out new interests, places, and things. These can go from being your enemy to being your friend and ally.

REPLACEMENT THERAPY

When hearing the words *replacement therapy* in regard to quitting, many will think immediately of nicotine replacement. While this may be essential to some more than to others, and definitely fits under the category, it is not the only type of replacement therapy you will have.

Consider this scenario: You have been at work for almost two and a half hours. Your first break is coming soon, and it is the one you spend with Charla on the back patio. You sit on the bench and talk about work and home, how the weekend was, or what current events are taking place in each other's life. You also smoke. Your body knows this

Write It Down! My Smoking Triggers

Turn to the chart on page 305 in the Appendix, and list your cravings to smoke, and what preceded those cravings, to help establish what some of your triggers may be. (If more convenient, you might want to hand copy the chart into your journal for easy reference as you work toward eliminating those cravings.)

Reviewing these lists can help you establish a pattern and consider replacement therapy.

is coming, and you can feel the desire building inside you. It is a physical craving your body recognizes, and you feel anxious and excited. The time comes, and you see Charla walking toward your desk. You grab your smokes, and the two of you walk out together to have a smoke. The cigarette helps you feel calm again, relaxed, and soon you are ready to go back to work.

Now consider this scenario: Again, you have been at work for the same two and a half hours. The same break is coming soon, and you usually spend it with Charla. You have quit smoking now, though, and being around her cigarette smoke makes your cravings unmanageable. You have a choice to make. You can stick with your usual routine, walk out with her, watch her smoke and talk to her, and try to resist the desire to smoke, and, if you succeed, you may feel even more anxious and nervous when you return after your break, which makes your break counterproductive. You struggle through your work, and just when you begin to recover from your morning break, it is time for lunch. The cycle starts again.

You will be faced with situations similar to this when you quit, and you could try this approach, or you could try some replacement therapy. What if you replaced your smoking break with Charla with a walk around the block? Or a visit to the other side of the building with a nonsmoking friend or acquaintance? Or what if you spoke with Charla and explained that you have quit, and ask her if she would mind doing something different? There are many options you could choose from to help you achieve success.

You might think of things that keep your hands busy. Avoid weight gain by chewing gum, eating carrot sticks, or sucking on something else that is shaped the same as your cigarettes, to keep your hands and mouth busy. This will ease your transition into a nonsmoking world.

Try new hobbies. Try to find something that will enable you to place your interests elsewhere and occupy your mind and hands when those cravings come. When you have identified your triggers, avoiding as many of them as possible will ease the number of cravings you have. But not all situations can be avoided. This is where a replacement for smoking that cigarette will prove to be beneficial.

SET A QUIT DATE AND FIND A SPONSOR

Now that you have decided to quit, identified your triggers, and considered some replacement therapies, you need to set a quit date. A quit date is a date you schedule to be the day of your last cigarette. It needs to be far enough away that you have enough time to become very aware of your triggers throughout the day, to organize some of your replacement therapies, and meet with your physician for nicotine replacement, if you want it. And one last thing—you need to find a support person or sponsor that you trust to help you.

After identifying who you would like this person to be, talk to him or her about becoming involved in your plan to quit. After the person agrees to be your sponsor, let him or her know what your triggers are, and what you are trying to avoid. Tell your sponsor about your replacement therapies, your nicotine replacements, and any other methods you expect to use to help you quit. Work with your sponsor to come up with some phrases you can use in difficult times and rehearse them so they are natural to you when the time comes to actually use them for real. Try these:

"I know I can do this."

"I am a strong person."

"I am a nonsmoker."

"I am a good example to those around me."

"I am healthy."

"I am taking care of my body."

"I am stronger than my cravings."

"I am loved."

"I can change myself."

"I can change my habits."

The more natural they are, the more likely you are to believe yourself when you say them. You can say these things silently to yourself, but you will feel different and get better results if you say them aloud so you can hear your voice reinforce the self-statement. Say it strongly and with conviction. Your brain will interpret your tone just as it does somebody else's, so your confidence in your statement does matter.

Let your sponsor know of the date of your last cigarette, and ask him or her to help you work through this and boost your efforts. Ask your sponsor to hold you responsible for what you are doing and the choices you are making.

Next, you get to make goals. Set beginning, intermediate, and advanced goals for yourself. This gives you something specific to work toward, as well as a reward to give yourself at the end of each goal. Start with something small, and move forward from there. Soon you will have the feeling of pride in yourself and your success. The reward will recognize your efforts from the outside, but the greatest change will take place inside you.

Write It Down! My Quitting Goals

Think about your short-term, medium-term, and advanced goals when it comes to quitting smoking. Write them down in the chart on page 305 in the Appendix. You might also want to copy these into your journal, to remind yourself to stick to them!

SIGN A QUITTING CONTRACT

A quitting contract is a simple promise to yourself and to your life that you will quit smoking. See page 306 in the Appendix for

> ### *Write It Down! My Quitting Contract and Quitting Calendar*
> Turn to page 306 in the Appendix to sign your quitting contract as witnessed by your sponsor. You may also want to buy a special calendar—a quitting calendar—so you can mark the days you've been smoke-free, as well as note when you've reached your goals. Alternatively, use the calendar on page 307 in the Appendix or create one in your journal and fill it in there.

a prototype of this agreement. Have your sponsor sign also, as a witness to your pledge to quit.

Now it's time to wait for your quit day to arrive, and brace yourself for a wild ride for a few days. It might be tough for a little while, but with your outlined plan, support center, replacement therapies, and rewards, you are ready to take it on and shine.

With your support in place, you'll be prepared to hit those withdrawals, setbacks, ornery moments, cravings, triumphs, changes, ultimate success, and rewards head on—with the little engine you are successfully driving up that impossible hill. Take it one hour, one day, one week at a time. Don't focus on the big picture but, instead, pieces of it. Don't hold onto old failures, if you have them. They don't matter. You are doing for yourself the single greatest thing you can do right now, and you deserve the success and rewards that will soon follow.

WITHDRAWAL

Nicotine is a powerful substance. Don't be surprised if you suffer from some type of withdrawal symptoms when you follow through on your choice to quit. *This is normal, and they will pass.* Be prepared for these symptoms by making yourself familiar with what they are and how you may feel. When you quit smoking, your lungs will produce excess mucus, and you will most likely cough more than usual for a little while. Do not let this alarm you! Your lungs are simply trying to cleanse themselves. It will pass. There are other things you may experience during your nicotine withdrawals. Watch for the following:

Mood swings	Irritability
Headaches	"Foggy" head
Low energy level	Coughing

Remind yourself and those around you that these things are only temporary, and that they are worth experiencing to reach the outcome. The reward will soon come. Try to keep yourself busy. Take a walk, play a game, or spend time with friends that support your efforts. Avoid spending time where smoking is taking place, to avoid the temptation to try "just one." Do things you enjoy doing, but try to choose activities that are not as strongly linked with your smoking habit as others might be.

It will be good to keep your hands occupied to distract you, so keep finger foods available. However, remember to make your choice of snacks healthy, low-fat snacks, such as crunchy apple slices and other fruits, carrots, celery and dip, granola, pretzels, popcorn, and low-fat cakes and cookies.

Remember, if you have tried this before and failed, it is okay. Don't carry that weight around with you, and don't doubt yourself this time. Take baby steps. Replace negative thoughts with positive self-statements. Keep your hands busy, stay away from people who are smoking, and replace activities that trigger your desire for a smoke with something new. Reinforce what you are trying to accomplish within yourself. This is not an easy thing to do, and requires a lot of lifestyle changes, but the rewards will come. You can do it!

WHAT IF YOU RELAPSE?

Inevitably, you may be wondering, "What if I relapse? What if I can't make it stick?" First, there are a couple of words and phrases you need to be familiar with. The first one is *setback*: a momentary return to a former frame of mind or behavior. It is a temporary thing. While it may take place more than once, it is something that can be resolved. And while it may not be easily overcome, and may take some dedication, it is not a total return to your previous state.

The second term you need to be familiar with is *relapse*: a return to your original habit. It is greater than a setback in that it is a complete surrender to your previous condition.

If you are a smoker, quitting may be something that you are all too familiar with. You may have quit several times, only to relapse, surrendering to the cravings and your old tendencies. If this is the case, you are not alone. What you need to understand is that you are combating a host of elements. First, you are combating addiction.

Addiction can be a monster to fight. The dictionary definition says it all: "The state of being enslaved to a habit or practice, or something that is psychologically or physically habit forming, such as narcotics, to such an extent that its cessation causes severe trauma."

In the case of smoking, nicotine causes a physical addiction. This can be helped with the use of pharmacologic agents, such as a nicotine patch or gum, or other smoking cessation drug therapies and step-down programs that can ease you through ending the nicotine dependence. Yet surprisingly enough, for many, this is not the most difficult thing to overcome.

Your life has actually been built around your habits. Quitting smoking is something that will alter the way your entire day may run. Think about it. Perhaps you are someone who has a smoke right after breakfast or on your way to work. Then you have your breaks at work, lunch, a possible commute home, dinner, after dinner smoke, evening, and bedtime. Perhaps you not only have scheduled smoke times but also have people you regularly smoke with and places where you light up. You may have your regular stops en route to your destinations that are traditionally where you get your cigarettes. As you can see, it is easy to understand why quitting affects your life so drastically, and why setbacks and relapse are so common for so many people. If you are one of the many who struggle to quit, even though your health may be declining and you struggle to breathe, it can be very difficult.

The good news is, you can do it. Think of it this way—millions of people have managed to successfully kick the habit. It has to be possible!

Even though it is difficult, and many things in your life will change, there are ways to quit that work. One of them will work for you.

Don't quit trying. If you have a setback, climb back on the saddle and continue the ride. Move forward. Don't let it discourage you to the point of giving up, but let it be something that pushes you forward. Having one puff or one cigarette doesn't mean you have to go back to your regular habit. Approach it from a positive outlook, and create and memorize positive self-statements to repeat to yourself when you don't reach your goals:

> "I may have had a setback today, but it is still less than I used to smoke, so I am still moving forward."
>
> "I am still strong and capable. I will do better tomorrow."
>
> "I can take this one day at a time. If I didn't do as well as I wanted today, I can still make it to the end."
>
> "I am successful."
>
> "I did it, just for today."

It is important for you to realize that one of the biggest mistakes you can make in your efforts is not forgiving yourself for failing. In regard to relapse, forgive yourself and try, try again. Become that "little engine that could" and continue to reinforce your successes and push yourself to your limits. Stretch beyond them. Remember, success isn't something that is won; it is something that is earned. You *can* do it. Love yourself. Forgive yourself. Keep fighting.

As Abraham Lincoln said, "Always bear in mind that your own resolution to succeed is more important than any other."

Choosing to quit smoking is such an incredible thing to do for yourself. It takes dedication and focus. Another thing that can also take dedication and focus can be your diet. Eating the correct food and the right combinations of foods can make a great difference on how you feel and perform. How is your diet? How can it be improved? The next step offers some great suggestions.

Choose Foods for Better Breathing

It's not what you say out of your mouth that determines your life, it's what you whisper to yourself that has the most power.

— ROBERT T. KIYOSAKI

Now that you know the importance of understanding how your own body works and how COPD affects it, isn't it time to properly fuel your machine? Did you know that the fuel you put in your body can help or hinder your efforts? Your respiratory system consists of muscles, and those muscles need nutrition to function. Your respiratory system is therefore greatly affected by the foods you choose. Moreover, when you don't get enough nutrients, it's disruptive and impairs *all* your organ systems and muscles. To compound the situation, disease can inhibit nutrient intake or alter metabolism, both of which can cause malnutrition.

Have you ever felt yourself falling victim to this: You are having a rough patch with regard to your breathing, you're tired of the feeling your meds leave in your mouth, and you might be a little depressed, or having trouble during your regular meals. Maybe the seasons are changing, there is pollen in the air that is causing you greater breathing difficulty, or any number of events may be taking place. Regardless of the cause, you're struggling and experiencing worsening symptoms for a day, a week, a month.

With this worsening of symptoms is the first step in this downward spiral and you're left feeling that it's harder to perform activities. With your aerobic capacity impaired, you begin to lose muscle strength. A decrease in muscular ability will occur after two weeks of decreased activity. Upon decreased muscle strength, you will again experience a worsening of symptoms. With this, malnutrition often follows because your metabolic rate increases, caused by your burning more calories breathing and the use of extra muscles to do so. This is known as the COPD Cycle of Malnutrition—similar to the COPD Downward Spiral (the anxiety-dyspnea cycle) you learned about in Step 6.

THE COPD CYCLE OF MALNUTRITION

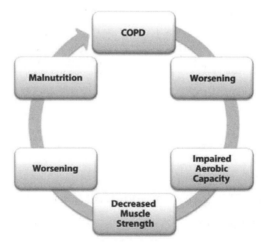

As you can see, halting this cycle is essential for your well-being. The cycle can be endless, unless you work to break it.

Malnutrition is not purely about the *quantity* of you eat food; it is possible to be overweight and yet malnourished. It is simply a state of being *improperly* nourished, such as from a diet full of processed foods instead of healthy ones. It can also be due to your not taking in enough nutrition to meet your body's daily demands and requirements. And malnutrition can occur more easily than you might think: You are burning extra calories each day just to breathe; meanwhile, it may be difficult for you to prepare food or eat due to weakness and fatigue, your meds (which may interfere with your ability to taste or smell, or otherwise adversely affect your appetite), or your oxygen (which can dry out your mouth). This cycle can be endless, unless you take steps to break it.

Let's talk for a moment about the deconditioning that can often accompany or follow this cycle. Now, you may have heard the term *deconditioning* before, outside the context of COPD. Your muscles, when used regularly during an exercise routine, retain "muscle memory" and tone for a period of two weeks' time. During prolonged periods of inactivity, the muscle tissues lose their muscle memory, and tone begins to diminish at a rapid rate. The strength and tone it took you a week to gain will be lost in two days' time. When your muscle size begins to shrink and tone is diminished, you may begin to decondition (to lose your overall physical fitness). People with chronic disease are at increased risk of deconditioning. Simply put, you need to feed your muscles, to keep up their strength.

In the following pages, you'll find some guidelines for a healthy diet. Your physician will also give you guidelines to follow regarding your disease and your nutritional needs. If your physician doesn't bring up the topic of diet, please don't hesitate to ask whether there are specific nutritional habits you need to practice each day, or whether you can be put in touch with a dietitian familiar with the needs of COPD patients. The advice in this section is not intended to replace the advice your health-care providers offer. However, it is up to each of us to self-advocate for our well-being. The power is in your hands to make healthy decisions.

First, let's take a look at the basic components of nutrition.

MACRONUTRIENTS: YOUR SOURCE OF ENERGY

Whether moving or resting, your body expends energy. You use energy to breathe, sleep, walk, talk, eat, and so forth. Macronutrients supply the body with energy requirements. You need to consume three kinds of macronutrients: carbohydrates, proteins, and fat.

Each of these macronutrients supplies the body with 4, 4, and 9 calories per gram, respectively. And while you probably hear the word *calorie* a lot, here's a quick explanation of why calories are crucial to you: A calorie is a measurement of heat that is used to indicate the amount of energy that a food will produce in the human body. The higher the calories, the more energy produced. What is important is to make sure the calories you take in are nutrient dense, meaning that they have vitamins and minerals that your body needs as opposed to a higher percentage of refined sugars and unhealthy fats (also known as empty calories).

Carbohydrates: There are two types of carbohydrates: simple and complex. Simple carbohydrates are found in refined sugars, such as those in candies, cakes, cookies, pies, pastries, milk, fruits, juices, sugary drinks, and other sweetened foods. A healthy diet for a person with chronic lung disease will include lesser quantities of these foods (we'll talk more about this in a few pages). Complex carbohydrates, on the other hand, which provide your body with healthy energy, are found in whole grains, vegetables, legumes, nuts, seeds, and fruits. These foods should make up 50 to 60 percent of your diet.

Protein: Protein is composed of nine essential and eleven nonessential amino acids. Consuming a varied diet with adequate calories each day provides the amino acids the body requires for building and maintaining muscle. Animal protein (meat, fish, dairy) varies slightly from vegetable protein; however, soy protein is almost identical to animal protein.

Many people try to stay away from meat, to avoid its fat and cholesterol content. Vegetarian or vegan diets can be healthy and beneficial in preventing and treating certain diseases, but if you choose to follow a diet that includes no animal products, it is essential to incorporate protein from soy, beans, and nuts as well as supplement the diet with vitamins B_{12} and D. A healthy halfway measure might be to ban red meat and high-fat dairy from your menu, while still consuming other forms of animal protein, such as chicken or fish.

Fats: Fat is the most concentrated source of calories in your diet. For this reason, a reduction in fat intake will ultimately show a reduction in caloric intake. Like carbs, there are different types of fat—some beneficial. The three types of natural fats are: saturated, monounsaturated, and polyunsaturated fatty acids. Trans fats, on the other hand, occur in very small amounts naturally but are chemically engineered for use in processed products.

Found mainly in animal products, **saturated fats** raise your body's cholesterol levels more than monounsaturated and polyunsaturated fatty acids do. These fats are solid at room temperature (an easy way to tell which kind of fat is which). Keep in mind that many foods that are high in saturated fats are also high in calories—such foods as fatty beef, pork, lard, cream, cheese, butter, and whole dairy products, to name a few. Many baked goods also contain saturated fats. A few plant oils that contain saturated fats include palm oil and coconut oil, but these do not contain cholesterol. It is a good idea to limit your intake of these fats— the American Heart Association recommends limiting your intake of saturated fats to only 5 to 6 percent of your daily caloric intake.

Healthier for you than saturated fats, **monounsaturated and polyunsaturated fatty acids**, a.k.a. the "good" fats, come from plants. Here's the difference between the two: Monounsaturated fatty acids, found in olive, canola, and nut-based oils, are the healthiest of all the fats, and are generally liquid at room temperature; they do not turn solid until slightly chilled. Polyunsaturated fatty acids are found in many vegetable oils, including safflower, sunflower, corn, soy and cottonseed oils. They are second best, as far as healthy fats go, but are also a little different than monounsaturated fats in that the omega-3 and omega-6 oils fall into this group. Flaxseeds, walnuts, some fatty fish (such as salmon and herring), pecans, Brazil nuts, and sesame oil all contain omega-3 and omega-6 oils, which are healthy for brain function, aid in the reduction of inflammation in your body, and lower your risk of heart disease.

Trans fats, on the other hand, are the worst kind of fat. For the most part man-made, they are formed in an industrial process in which hydrogen is added to vegetable oil, causing the oil to become solid at room temperatures. These fats are found in many baked goods, snacks, fried foods, refrigerated doughs, margarine, and creamers. Look for the term *partially hydrogenated* on ingredient labels so you can avoid it.

Ideally, no more than 25 to 35 percent of caloric intake should come from fats. That amount should be distributed among the three fatty acids: less than 10 percent saturated fatty acids, 10 percent polyunsaturated, and 10 to 15 percent monounsaturated. You should avoid trans fats as much as possible. If your condition worsens to the point where you find yourself underweight, struggling to keep weight on, or trying to gain weight, healthy fats are the first thing you want to focus on while consuming your extra calories because of the way they are metabolized in the body. It is much better to concentrate on eating extras of these foods as well as proteins, instead of increasing carbohydrate consumption.

MICRONUTRIENTS: KEEPING YOUR CELLS RUNNING

Micronutrients do not provide energy but are nonetheless essential to human health and survival. They include vitamins, minerals, and other bioactive chemicals that affect your tissue and can be found in the foods you eat. Height, weight, activity level, your body's growth state (infants and teens, pregnancy), surgery, trauma, disease, infection or inflammation, fever, and medications are some factors that can influence your nutritional needs. Micronutrients include vitamins, minerals, antioxidants, phytonutrients, and more.

Vitamins and Minerals

Vitamins and minerals are essential and play key roles in muscle contraction as well as fluid and acid base balance. Half of the American population (and probably you) takes micronutrient supplements, many of which are prescribed. Something most people don't know is that when your diet is optimal, routine use of nutritional supplements is not usually necessary! You can usually get everything you need from readily available foods. The best way for you to obtain the recommended levels of micronutrients is by eating a healthy diet full of fresh fruits and plenty of vegetables; lean protein found in beans, chicken, fish, and wild game; and plenty of grains and fiber; while restricting your intake of refined sugars and other simple carbohydrates, and of processed foods. In short, stick to clean foods. Review the menu ideas on pages 225–233 for some sample meal plans that include these foods.

Vitamins

Vitamins are either fat soluble or water soluble, meaning they are absorbed in either the fat or water in your body. One thing to be wary of is the use of nonprescription, fat-soluble supplements, unless you have consulted with your physician. Let me tell you why. Fat-soluble vitamins, such as vitamins A, D, E, and K, reside in your body's fatty tissues and liver to be stored until needed by your body. This storage, in excess, can lead to problems because as they are stored, they can also accumulate to an unhealthy degree.

Water-soluble vitamins, such as vitamin C, thiamine (B_1), riboflavin (B_2), niacin (B_3), pantothenic acid (B_5), biotin (B_7), folic acid (B_9), cobalamin (B_{12}), and tryptophan, are not generally stored in your body and are therefore not as much of a risk for you to take. They work best when you take just what you need each day. When you take water-soluble vitamins, your body will absorb what it needs and excrete the rest, thus the need to replenish these vitamins each day. However, just because excess is eliminated each day doesn't mean you can take as much as you like. It is still best to not exceed the upper limits of each, as too much vitamin C has been known to cause kidney stones, too much niacin can cause flushing, too much vitamin B_6 has been shown to cause problems with nerves, and so on. If you do decide to take supplements, be sure to consult with your health-care provider.

Minerals

Minerals are also required by your body for healthy function. There are minerals that your body needs each day. The good news is that just like the other items listed here, these minerals can be found in the healthy, whole foods that you eat, and by eating a healthy diet you are likely to feed your cells the nutrients they need and avoid mineral deficiencies. (If you do suffer from mineral deficiencies, your doctor can find that out by running a blood panel, and he or she may prescribe mineral supplements, if needed.) So, what minerals do you need each day? Keep in mind that while we are discussing necessary minerals, the actual amount we need each day will vary depending on age, sex, and level of health or sickness. Your physician and/or dietician can help you determine what exactly your body needs.

There are a few major minerals the body needs. They include calcium, chloride, magnesium, phosphorus, potassium, sodium, and sulfur. There are also trace minerals the body needs. They include iron, iodine, cobalt, chromium, selenium, copper, fluorine, manganese, molybdenum, and zinc. We will focus on all the major minerals and some of the trace minerals. While there are currently no conclusive studies on minerals and COPD, it would be good to be aware of these minerals and where you can find them for your overall health.

Calcium is the first major mineral our body needs. It is required for developing and maintaining strong bones and teeth. Most of the calcium in our body is actually stored in our bones and teeth. You may have heard the words *calcium* and *magnesium* heard together. That is because calcium needs magnesium, as well as phosphorus and vitamins D and K, for adequate and proper absorption. Calcium is important to avoid such conditions as osteoporosis, hypertension (high blood pressure), and high cholesterol. Dietary sources of calcium include dairy products, dark leafy greens as well as broccoli, oysters and sardines, and almonds.

Chloride is another mineral that we need for optimal function. Chloride is an electrolyte that works in conjunction with sodium and carbon dioxide, to maintain the acid base balance in the body as well as help to maintain a proper balance of fluids in our cells. Fluid follows these electrolytes in and out of our cells. If you have high levels of chloride, you may be experiencing dehydration or respiratory alkalosis (a medical condition that results in too high a pH in the blood); if you have depleted chloride, you may be experiencing congestive heart failure or vomiting. Dietary sources of chloride include celery, olives, salt, and tomatoes.

Magnesium is another essential mineral necessary for the healthy growth of bones and teeth as well as for the normal function of our nervous system and muscle cells. It is necessary for the electrolytes in our bodies to function properly, oxidizes fatty acids, prevents the formation of bad cholesterol, and helps activate amino acids. Too little can cause sleepiness and muscle spasms, and too much can cause low blood pressure or cardiac arrest. Dietary sources of magnesium include halibut, white beans, soy, whole grains, dark green vegetables such as spinach, and cashews.

Phosphorus is another mineral with responsibility for building strong teeth and bones. It is the second most abundant mineral in the body, next to calcium. It helps in filtering out waste from the kidneys and also helps our body store and then use energy. It is useful in cell growth and repair, and can be found in milk and meats. If your diet includes healthy levels of calcium, you are getting healthy amounts of phosphorus, as well.

Potassium is used in muscle-to-nerve communication as well as in moving nutrients into cells in conjunction with removing waste from the cells. Kidney failure and blood transfusions are the most common causes of elevated potassium, while vomiting and extended or chronic diarrhea or the use of diuretics are cause for depleted levels of potassium. It can be found in bananas, pears, tomato juice, sweet potatoes, pumpkin, turkey, peaches, and grapes. You will also find it in some dairy products, such as ice cream or yogurt.

We talked about the fluids in our cells following the chloride. Well, an even more important mineral in that job is sodium. Sodium is primarily responsible and absolutely necessary for the human body to have, for it to maintain fluid balance. It is also responsible for transmitting nerve impulses and is an important player in muscle contraction and relaxation. Too much sodium can lead to such problems as heart disease, high blood pressure (which can cause stroke), and kidney disease. Sodium is easily found in condiments and processed foods, such as canned soup, and is easy to get enough of. (If you have ever had to limit your sodium intake due to fluid retention, you will understand how easily accessible sodium is, and how difficult it can really be to remove it from your diet.)

Iodine is a trace mineral required for proper mental and physical development. It is utilized in the conversion of energy for our nerves, muscles, skin, hair, and teeth as well as assists in the repairing of damaged tissues. Too little iodine will contribute to skin problems, insomnia, fatigue, and weight gain. It can be found in high levels in seafood. It is always a good idea to buy iodized salt for your table salt to assist in the availability of iodine.

Iron is necessary for building muscle and maintaining healthy blood. You have probably heard that iron is necessary for oxygen delivery. This is because the hemoglobin that oxygen molecules attach themselves to are actually attached to the iron molecules in your blood. For this reason, if you are low on iron (anemic), you will have a harder time oxygenating.

Dietary sources of iron include clams, organs meats such as liver, oysters, soybeans, iron-fortified cereals, pumpkin seeds, beans, and spinach.

Zinc is needed for a healthy immune system, and that is so important when you have an underlying condition, such as chronic lung disease. It is also important for the production of certain hormones and healthy skin. Seafood can be zinc rich, as well as spinach and cashews, and . . . dark chocolate.

Chromium is another mineral that our body needs. It is responsible for the function of glucose, which is responsible for making sure every cell in our body gets the energy it needs when it is needed. As long as your diet includes plenty of whole grains and vegetables, you should be getting enough chromium, but you can find it in apples, bananas, and green peppers as well as liver, beef, chicken, and eggs.

Copper is another trace mineral. Its primary function is to assist in the absorption of iron, which we already know is a must have for our red blood cells. It is also utilized to build skin, bones, and other tissues and is important for the immune, nervous, and cardiovascular systems. Copper serves a dual role as a great antioxidant, which is described in the next section.

Manganese is a trace mineral that is used to keep bones and skin healthy but also has an important function in protecting cells from free radicals, also described in the next section.

Antioxidants

Antioxidants are natural substances, commonly found in brightly colored fruits and vegetables, which help protect cells from damage caused by compounds called free radicals. Free radicals are unstable molecules that are a by-product of metabolism, meaning they occur naturally, often during cell death. They are free hydrogen ions that are searching for a positive balance to adhere to. During this process, they essentially bounce off tissues in your body and cause damage each time they hit.

Oxidation is an interaction between oxygen molecules and other substances. It occurs in everything from the metal on your car to the tissues in your body. It is what is happening when an apple or banana begins to turn brown after you peel it. Because the process of oxidation contributes to cell death, it can increase free radicals.

You might be wondering why this is important to you and how it pertains to COPD. Oxidation is what causes the destruction of the lung's air sacs, or alveoli. These, remember, are the area of gas exchange in your lungs. It's where the oxygen enters the blood and the carbon dioxide leaves the blood.

Your lungs, since they are open to the outside world, are subject to oxidants both from the outside world (such as cigarette smoke or pollution) as well as inside your body (released from cells). Oxidative stress is something that occurs when there is an imbalance between oxidants and antioxidants, caused by an overabundance of oxidants or a lack of antioxidants.

Antioxidants are proven to help stabilize and remove free radicals from our body. The most well-known antioxidants are vitamins C and E and beta-carotene. Studies are currently being done on the efficacy of antioxidants, and their role in boosting our immune system and preventing cancer. Lung disease patients who consume a diet rich in antioxidants tend to have better lung function than do those whose diet does not include antioxidants. Consuming fruits and vegetables can improve your ventilatory function, and slow or decrease the risks of COPD.

Phytochemicals

Phytochemicals are naturally occurring compounds that are found in plants, such as fruits and vegetables. While these compounds actually exist to protect the plant, recent research has found that may be protective for humans, as well. They are nonessential nutrients, meaning

Anti-Up!

According to the US Department of Agriculture, here are the top antioxidant-rich foods to include in your diet. Many of these are found in our sample menus on pages 221–222.

Apples, Gala, Granny Smith, or Red Delicious	Cranberries	Peppers
	Currant, red	Pineapple
	Fish	Plums
Artichoke hearts	Flaxseed	Pomegranates
Avocados	Garlic	Potatoes, russet
Beets	Ginger	Prunes
Blackberries	Green tea	Raspberries
Blueberries	Kale	Rosemary extract
Cabbage	Kelp	Spinach
Carrots	Mushrooms	Strawberries
Cherries, sweet	Olives	Turnip greens
Chocolate, dark	Olive oil	Tomato products
Cloves, ground	Oranges	Turmeric
Collard greens	Pecans	Walnuts

they are not required to sustain life but they can be beneficial to overall health. There are over a thousand presently known phytochemicals. In natural foods, they are responsible for much of the color, such as the deep purple of blueberries, or distinctive smells, such as that of garlic. They can be found in most natural foods but are not present in processed foods, refined sugars, or alcohols.

Most phytochemicals contain antioxidant properties to combat oxidative stress and fight certain types of cancers. They have been shown to buffer menopausal symptoms and reduce osteoporosis, contain antibacterial properties, and reduce the incidence of infection by binding to human cell walls and inhibiting pathogens from adhering to the same walls. Sounds like pretty good stuff to have hanging out in our cells, right?

TWO MORE KEY DIETARY COMPONENTS

Along with macro- and micronutrients, antioxidants, and phytochemicals, a couple more things that are important to include in your diet—fiber and fluids.

Fiber

Although dietary fiber is not a nutrient—it's an indigestible carbohydrate—it does play many important roles. There are two types of dietary fiber: soluble and insoluble. Insoluble fiber is found in whole grains, nuts, seeds, and some vegetables. Soluble fibers are found in fruits, fruit skins, oats, barley, and some vegetables. Fiber helps absorb water in the gastrointestinal (GI) tract, regulate your GI tract, reduce constipation and irritable bowel syndrome, regulate cholesterol and glucose levels, and help prevent cancer and diverticular disease. The recommended amount of fiber for the average adult is 25 grams per day.

Fluids

Drinking enough fluids is vital to maintain good health. Adults should consume at least 2 liters (8 cups) of fluid per day to prevent dehydration. Depending on your activity level, you may need more. Sources of fluids include water; other healthy beverages, such as fruit and vegetable juices and tea; prepared gelatin; ices, sorbets, and ice creams; soups, and anything else that is liquid at room temperature. As we age, we lose our sense of thirst. For this reason, those who are elderly or very active should intentionally consume fluids to prevent dehydration. We excrete fluid through respirations, sweating, and urine. Dehydration can affect your mucus viscosity (thickness), the ability to mobilize the mucus in your lungs, as well as the (fluid) levels in your body.

Some people have a difficult time drinking water. Adding freshly squeezed lemon juice to your water can improve the flavor and also has a second, really great benefit of improving your body's pH. Lemon juice helps neutralize your pH, which is better for overall health, fosters an environment that contributes to healthy cells, and stabilizes your entire system. So many benefits for such a small change! And remember, you can add this to every glass of water or just a few. Your choice.

Although most people can safely consume 8 to 16 cups of fluid per day, be sure to check with your physician on exactly how much fluid is safe for you, as some patients may have fluid restrictions depending on their health conditions. As a COPD patient, stay away from carbonated beverages (sodas and seltzers) as they increase your carbon dioxide levels, which interfere with your breathing patterns and make things more difficult for you.

NUTRITION FOR BETTER BREATHING

As a lung patient, your nutritional needs are special and maintaining a healthy weight is *essential.* You may have noticed that preparing meals may be more challenging than it used to be, but healthy habits are more important now than ever before. It may be difficult to fix a healthy meal, or even more difficult to eat it. Some symptoms that make it more difficult to eat and cook may be the following:

Dyspnea (difficulty breathing), which can lead to trouble chewing and/ or swallowing

Chronic mouth breathing, which can cause changes in your ability to taste

Coughing, which can interfere with eating

Fatigue

Excess mucus production

Medication side effects

Morning headaches, causing breakfast difficulties

COPD is a disease that affects the lungs, but it can have consequences for your entire body. There are several reasons nutrition management is essential in chronic lung disease. It is best for an ideal body weight to be maintained. If you carry extra weight, make changes in your lifestyle and diet to lose it, but one thing that is important to prevent is the unwanted weight loss that often accompanies severe COPD because patients that fall into that category typically do not have the weight to lose. It can become a balancing act for lung patients to maintain sufficient nutrition to stay at a healthy weight once this starts happening. As discussed, malnutrition is a big concern for anyone with lung disease. Malnutrition can adversely affect breathing by reducing the strength and function of the respiratory system, as well as skeletal muscles. Malnutrition can also increase susceptibility to infection, and lower exercise capacity. Patients must maintain their energy balance in spite of their increased caloric needs.

If you are overweight, safely losing excess weight is important, as unnecessary poundage can make it more difficult to breathe. Belly weight can hinder the ability of your diaphragm to descend, lessening the space your lungs have for expansion.

A healthy diet can also lead to better breathing on the molecular level, specifically with regard to carbon dioxide. A diet too high in carbohydrates, especially the refined sugars you will find in cakes, candies, cookies, breads, and so on, as well as soda and other sweetened beverages, can lead to excess carbon dioxide, which is a by-product of metabolism. This excessive carbon dioxide is usually expelled through the lungs. Patients with chronic lung disease have an impaired ability to take in oxygen and eliminate carbon dioxide. This inability for gas exchange increases your ventilatory demands, and your lungs must work harder to excrete the excess carbon dioxide.

Let's return to my patient, Linda. As she progressed through this program and her ability to move increased and her diet changed, she lost 30 pounds of excess weight, then gained 10 pounds of muscle through strength training. She had the opportunity (as she referred to it) to buy a whole new wardrobe but, more important, felt, moved, and was breathing better!

More About Carbon Dioxide (CO_2)

No one ever likes to say no to cookies and cake, but consuming refined sugars is something to avoid, especially if you have COPD. When sugars are metabolized in your body, they break down to form excess carbon dioxide, and your respiratory rate will increase to expel that excess CO_2 from your blood. You may have even noticed this happening to you.

As CO_2 shifts the acid-base balance of your blood, one of the best ways your body has to regulate its levels of carbon dioxide is through breathing: Messages are sent from receptors monitoring the CO_2 levels in your blood to your brain, which triggers your diaphragm to breathe either faster or slower to get your carbon dioxide level back to where it needs to be.

As a chronic lung patient, your having to breathe faster due to increased levels of carbon dioxide can be very difficult to deal with. Air trapping occurs because the tiny airways adjacent to your air sacs (alveoli) open and close depending upon the pressures around them. As your respiratory rate increases, the pressure changes within your lungs faster and more frequently. If your air sacs don't have the elasticity they used to, they aren't doing their job to help move the air out of your lungs, and air can get stuck in an air sac. This is air trapping. When this occurs several times in multiple sacs, the accumulated "stale" air makes it more difficult for you to breathe because it leaves less room in your lungs for fresh air. This compounds the situation, making it even more difficult to breathe. It can also put you at risk for placing extra work on your heart as you work harder to breathe.

Unfortunately, carbonated drinks cause the same problem as sugar. If you pay attention, you will notice that you feel a shortness of breath or an increased respiratory rate after eating excessive sweets or the drinking carbonated beverages, such as soda or seltzer. So, before you partake, ask yourself: "Is this cookie, piece of cake, candy, or drink worth all that difficulty for the next several hours?"

COPD and Excess Salt

Another issue is salt intake. We talked about how sodium helps move fluid into and out of your cells. Your body is, in large part, water. Water follows salt in and out of the cells in your body. If you eat too much salt, you will find you are retaining more water. For some, this isn't a huge problem; but for others, it creates difficulty on many levels. If you are now or have ever been on sodium restrictions, you understand what we are talking about. Your fingers, feet, or ankles may swell. The really hard thing about COPD and water retention is that a buildup of water in your blood can leak into your air sacs. This can make for difficult breathing. Even if it doesn't leak directly into your lungs and remains primarily in the tissues, that water retention can still interrupt your breathing patterns by constricting your diaphragm movement and causing inflammation in your tissues. Whichever way you look at it, it doesn't add up to be in your favor and is something worth monitoring. To reduce your risk of water retention, you'll want to limit salt intake to 1,500 mg per day or whatever your physician recommends.

COPD and Caffeine

You'll also want to limit your caffeine intake. Caffeine creates feelings of alertness in our body because it increases the activity of our nervous system, resulting in an increase in our heart and respiratory rates. Now that you have learned how refined sugars and soda affect your breathing, by increasing your respiratory rate to eliminate CO_2, you understand how this can cause air trapping and know the trouble that creates. With the intake of high levels of caffeine "waking up" our nervous system and forcing it to work faster, our body naturally increases the rate at which we breathe so as to deliver more oxygen to our tissues. This, just like the increased breathing rate we have already discussed, can cause air trapping. This can put excess stress on the heart and lungs and cause muscle fatigue and irritability, as well. In addition to these issues, there is also a risk of caffeine interactions with some of the medications you may be prescribed, and this is worth checking with your pharmacist about. One thing to keep in mind is that you may experience headaches or symptoms of withdrawal, such as fatigue, irritability, and nervousness if you stop drinking caffeine, so taper yourself off carefully and cut back at a rate that will not cause you additional discomfort.

Gas-Causing Foods

Unfortunately, lots of foods—even healthy ones—can cause excess gas. This can, not only cause discomfort, but also may restrict your diaphragm's ability to expand, which will affect your ability to breathe. (Another reason for having gas is swallowed air. This can be avoided by eating slowly, chewing with your mouth closed, not using drinking straws or chewing gum, and not gulping your food.)

If gas is a problem for you, here is a list of foods to consider limiting in your diet:

Alcohol	Melons
Beer	Milk
Beans (dried)	Mushrooms
Broccoli	Nuts
Cabbage	Onions (raw)
Carbonated beverages	Peas
Cauliflower	Peppers
Cheeses (strong)	Popcorn
Chewing gum	Radishes
Corn	Spicy foods
Cucumbers	Sweet potatoes
Eggs	Turnips
Lentils	Wheat germ
Lettuce	Yogurt

Remember, different foods affect different people in different ways. Please use discretion in choosing which foods to eliminate so as to not ignore your nutritional needs. With the exception of alcohol, beer, and carbonated beverages, the foods listed are healthy if you can tolerate them. Consult your physician if you have extensive questions regarding which foods would be best for you to eliminate, or schedule an appointment with a registered dietitian to address your specific dietary needs.

SOME GENERAL GUIDELINES

Foods and Beverages to Avoid

- Foods high in simple carbohydrates, such as cakes, cookies, and other packaged items that contain refined sugars
- Soda, which is full of carbon dioxide as well as sugar
- Excessive salt or caffeine
- Foods that cause gas and bloating; a full abdomen can hinder your ability to breathe

Cooking Tips

- **Remember: If you wear oxygen, do not use a gas stove or work over a barbecue grill. Open flames and sparks are not friends with oxygen and can cause a fire.**
- Use an electric stove, oven, toaster oven, or microwave.
- Choose foods that are easy to eat.
- Bake meats as opposed to frying and use a steamer for vegetables, simplifying your meal preparation.
- Prepare what you can at the times of day when you have the most energy.

Eating Tips

- Chew foods thoroughly to help you avoid swallowing air while eating.
- Eat several smaller meals instead of fewer large ones, which may help with breathlessness.

- Eat slowly and carefully so as to avoid aspirating your food. This can cause coughing, which will wear you out and can negatively affect your ability to complete your meal and get the nourishment you need.
- Eat while sitting up. Use good posture.
- If you are on oxygen, wear your cannula while eating to ensure oxygen remains available.
- Drink liquids at the end of your meal to avoid feeling full.
- Make meals enjoyable by making it a social event when you can.
- Rest before and after meals.

TOP 10 FOODS FOR COPD PATIENTS TO EAT EVERY DAY

- Whole grains
- Plenty of vegetables, especially dark leafy greens; select those that are nongassy for you
- Lean protein, such as chicken, fish, and eggs
- Legumes
- Nuts–the perfect high-calorie snack
- 2% milk or almond milk
- Greek yogurt (unless you produce excessive mucus and it increases your symptoms)
- Fruits
- Vitamin and mineral supplements (according to your doctor's orders)
- And, of course, plenty of water—remember, you can add fresh lemon juice to any water you are drinking.

WHAT TO EAT: SAMPLE MENUS

For some people, rather than eating three large meals a day, it's easier to break them down into five or six smaller meals. As mentioned in other parts of this book, an overly full stomach can contribute to respiratory difficulties just through simple anatomy: When your stomach is too full, your diaphragm movement is limited. Since your diaphragm is the major breathing muscle, this makes for difficulty in breathing and shortness of breath. Also, because of the extra energy you are using to breathe, you may need up to 500 extra calories per day to sustain your energy levels (you may be burning up to ten times what a healthy person will use to breathe!). This doesn't mean you should fill up on cakes and candies, however. Remember, foods with simple carbohydrates (sugars) will elevate your carbon dioxide levels, which will cause shortness of breath. The trick is to eat small, nutrient-dense meals that will help you maintain your energy and remove the barrier with your diaphragm that large meals cause.

For some people, especially when eating becomes such a chore, it can be difficult to decide what to eat. For this reason, I have included a few sample menus for you to use as ideas, follow if you would like, and even pick through and take the parts you like, substitute the parts you don't, and do with it what you choose. These are, however, only ideas for you to pull from. This is not a diet that is directed toward any one person, or any one diagnosis, it is simply healthy choices to draw from. If you have severe COPD, and as mentioned earlier, your physician has you on strict diet limitations or directions, please be sure to follow the recommendations of your physician or dietitian.

Patients with COPD will burn more calories breathing than when their lungs were healthy. For many patients, 40 to 70 percent of COPD sufferers, unintentional weight loss takes place. For this reason it is important to remember and calculate your caloric intake and output. You can count as a general rule that you will burn anywhere from 500 to 1000 extra calories per day breathing (a person with normal lung function will burn approximately 100 calories per day breathing). These calories burned will increase as your work of breathing increases. This is why your diet will need to change in order for you to maintain a healthy weight. As your breathing becomes more labored, your caloric intake will need to increase to meet demand and to supply you with enough energy to breathe effectively. You may end up increasing your caloric intake by as many as 1,500 calories per day at some point. When eating is already exhausting and difficult, this can really be taxing. Here are some sample menus composed of a good combination of healthy carbs, proteins, and fats complete with micronutrients, antioxidants, fiber, and fluid.

Breakfast

- 1 egg, 1 piece of whole-grain toast, 1 ounce of sliced turkey topped with avocado slices, ½ cup of fresh fruit, 4 ounces of fruit juice of choice, 4 ounces of milk of choice
- 1 cup of vanilla Greek yogurt topped with ½ cup of granola, ½ large grapefruit, ½ banana, 4 ounces of fruit juice of choice
- 1 cup of oatmeal or whole-grain cereal, ½ cup of blueberries, ½ cup of cottage cheese, 4 ounces of fruit juice of choice, 4 ounces of milk of choice

Lunch

- Green salad (any size): Mixed lettuce greens, spinach, and kale, plus your choice of other vegetables (such as beets, carrots, celery, peas, tomatoes, or other favorites), proteins (such as kidney or black beans, chicken, turkey, quinoa, or boiled egg), cheese (preferably white), black olives, seeds or nuts (such as sunflower seeds, pecans, almonds, or walnuts), dressed with freshly squeezed lemon or lime juice or 2 tablespoons of olive oil and vinegar dressing, and a whole wheat roll
- 3 ounces of grilled chicken, 1 cup of steamed, nongassy vegetables, ½ cup of cooked brown rice, ½ cup of fresh raspberries or blueberries
- Sandwich on whole-grain bread: 2 ounces of sliced turkey, 2 pieces of crisp romaine lettuce, 2 slices of tomato, 1 slice of provolone cheese, 1 teaspoon of mayonnaise, 1 teaspoon of mustard, a small bunch of bean sprouts, and sliced black olives, with 1 medium-size dill pickle and 2 ounces of potato chips on the side

Dinner

- Vegetable Beef Soup: Brown 1 pound of ground beef or beef chunks in a skillet, drain away the fat, and place the meat in a slow cooker. Add 16 ounces of tomato or vegetable juice, 2 carrots (sliced), 2 celery stalks (sliced), 3 potatoes (your choice, cubed), 1 cup of fresh green beans, and 1 cup each of broccoli and cauliflower (sliced into small florets). Simmer for 4 hours on LOW. Serve with 1 slice of whole-grain toast. Yield: 8 (1-cup) servings
- 3 ounces of roast beef, prepared your favorite way, ½ cup of mashed potatoes with a small amount of butter or gravy, 1 cup of fresh steamed vegetables, side salad of fresh vegetables, 1 slice of whole-grain bread, and 1 cup of milk of choice or lemon water
- 2 ounces of grilled salmon garnished with fresh lemon juice, ½ cup of cooked brown rice, 1 cup of steamed vegetables, and a side salad of fresh vegetables, served with a whole-grain roll and 1 cup of lemon water

Snacks, a.k.a. Mini Meals

- 4 celery stalks (cut into sticks) or 1 Gala, Red Delicious, or Granny Smith apple (sliced), plus ½ cup of peanut or almond butter, for dipping
- Protein shake made with 8 ounces of milk of choice, juice, or water
- ½ cup of cottage cheese plus 1 pear (sliced)
- 4 Protein Balls: To make, mix together 2 cups of rolled oats, 1 cup of shredded coconut, 1 cup of peanut butter, 1 cup of local honey, ¼ cup of flaxseeds, and ½ cup of chocolate chips or raisins until well blended, then form into 1-inch balls and freeze for about an hour. Refrigerate until eaten. Yield: 24 balls
- 2 cheese sticks (mozzarella), ½ cucumber (sliced), 10 to 15 black or green olives
- ½ cup of edamame, plus 6 cooked, chilled shrimp with ¼ cup of cocktail sauce
- Fruit smoothie made with frozen fruit: blueberries, raspberries, or sweet cherries, and Greek yogurt
- Orange Creamsicle smoothie

- ½ cup of pecans, walnuts, brazil nuts, cashews, or almonds
- ½ to 1 avocado (sliced)
- 2 boiled eggs

INSTEAD OF THIS	CHOOSE THIS
Soda	Fresh lemon water or fruit or vegetable juice
Fried chicken	Grilled chicken
Potato chips	Cucumber slices sprinkled with salt or apple chips
Sugary breakfast cereals	Whole-grain, iron and calcium-fortified cereals
Cookies	Fresh fruit slices and yogurt fruit dip or protein balls
Quesadilla	Chicken and shrimp fajitas with guacamole
Candy bar	Celery sticks with peanut butter
French fries	Apple slices or carrot sticks
White rice	Brown rice or quinoa
White bread	Whole grains
Soft-shell taco	Taco salad with dark leafy greens and veggies
White flour pasta	Whole wheat pasta
Cake	Cottage cheese and fruit
Chip dip	Hummus
Candy	Fruit leather or nuts

DIET AND SPECIAL NEEDS

Chronic disease can sometimes cause malnutrition and COPD is no exception to this rule. Due to the excessive exertion to simply breathe, paying special attention to the contents of your diet is especially important. For example, using the listed sample menus you will have a well-balanced, healthy diet full of protein, complex carbohydrates, fats, and micronutrients. This is a great base to your nutrition plan but will sometimes need to be altered to fit your specific needs. Let's look at a couple of situations in which this may apply but remember: Good nutrition doesn't have to be difficult!

Infection

If an infection or exacerbation occurs, you may need to increase your fluids to remain hydrated and increase your calories or adjust the method in which you get them in order to give your body enough energy to heal. A good way to do both of these would be to do the following:

- Include Ensure or Boost into your diet to supplement your intake and/or calories
- Include juices or extra fruit and vegetables
- Reduce intake of nutrient deficient foods (high calorie, low nutrition– think candy, cakes, soda)
- Increase low fat protein sources such as poultry or fish

Weight Management

For some patients in later stages of the disease, weight loss becomes what can seem to be a losing battle but there are tricks to help you win this war! For example, this can become your opportunity to really enjoy eating the foods you like best. For some, taste buds are not as "tasty" as they used to be and food can lack the luster and attraction it used to have because the taste isn't there, the enjoyment is reduced. For this, try to enjoy things such as

- Ice cream
- Whole milk
- Whole milk cheese
- Yogurt and granola
- Puddings
- Custards
- Peanut butter
- Bread sticks with cheese sauce
- Alfredo sauce and pastas
- Popcorn with extra butter
- Bagels and cream cheese

- Replacing milk on your cereal with half and half
- Including dips with your fruits and veggies
- Eating nuts
- Fruit smoothies with a protein supplement

You can also add calories to your diet by adding powdered milk to things like

- Mashed potatoes
- Sauces
- Hot cereal
- Gravies
- Puddings
- Casseroles

You can add extra eggs to things like meatloaf and casseroles and add extra jam, honey, and syrup to foods like cereal, toast, and granola.

Don't be afraid to be creative and add those extra calories you may have spent years trying to avoid! Just as little changes in eliminating them can lead to weight loss, adding them here and there can add essential calories you so desperately need right now. Making these simple changes can increase your daily caloric intake by hundreds of calories each day. Your doctor may also prescribe a nutritional supplement to help you maintain a healthy weight and increase your caloric intake.

RECIPES

Here are a few favorite meal ideas you can use to add extra calories to your diet.

Breakfast

Breakfast is an easy time to get carb overload—so watch yourself. Focus on protein-heavy foods to give you strength and to sustain healthy blood glucose levels and allow you to perform the required activities of your morning. Remember, you can also eat something simple such as a boiled egg and fresh fruit, too!

WHOLE GRAIN IN A BOWL

SERVES 1

Put your rice cooker to good use in making you a warm, hearty breakfast for a great kick start to your day!

  ½ cup wild rice
  ½ cup rolled oats
  ½ cup farina wheat cereal
  2 tablespoons packed brown sugar
  ⅓ cup favorite dried fruit
  Milk to taste

Place all ingredients in a rice cooker prior to going to bed at night. Close the cooker and program it to turn on and cook your Whole Grain in a Bowl for 50 minutes prior to waking up.

GREEK GRANOLA ON THE GO

SERVES 1

This is a simple, nutritious, and great on-the-go breakfast!

  ½ cup granola
  1 serving (8 ounces) vanilla Greek yogurt
  1 teaspoon honey to taste
  Favorite fruit

Place all ingredients in glass jar with a lid, top with favorite fruit, and store for up to 5 days for a quick, nutritious breakfast on the go.

AVOCADO BREAKFAST EGGS

SERVES 1

This hearty breakfast combines beneficial fats with proteins and carbs for a delicious, healthy way to start your day.

3 eggs
¼ cup milk
¼ cup chopped ham or turkey
Oil for pan
1 chopped green onion
⅛ chopped green pepper
¼ cup spinach
½ small tomato
¼ cup grated cheese
¼ avocado

In a small bowl, beat the eggs and milk until combined. Add oil to a medium-sized skillet and place it over medium heat. When the pan is warm, pour in the egg mixture so it coats the bottom of the pan. Cook the eggs until starting to firm, place ham and veggies (except avocado) inside egg. Remove to plate and top with cheese and sliced avocado.

Lunch

DELICIOUS GRILLED CHEESE

MAKES 1 SANDWICH

Sometimes simplest is tastiest! There's nothing quite like a homemade grilled cheese.

Butter

2 slices of your favorite bread

Mayonnaise to taste

Oil for pan

2 slices of whole milk cheese

2 slices of Monterey Jack Cheese

½ avocado, sliced

½ tomato, sliced

Heavily butter both slices of bread. If you are using mayo, spread that on one of the slices. Heat a medium-sized skillet or grill pan to medium heat. Add oil. Place one slice of bread, buttered side down, in the pan, and top with cheeses, avocado, and tomato. Place the top slice. Cook over medium heat until the cheese starts to melt; flip and cook until the cheese is fully melted.

HOMEMADE GUACAMOLE

SERVES 1

This easy guac is a great with tortilla chips or used as garnish. It's delicious served with eggs!

1 ripe avocado, smashed

½ tomato, diced

¼ white onion, diced

Pepper to taste

Mix all ingredients together. Best if eaten right away.

HAM AND CREAM CHEESE ROLL

MAKES 1 ROLL

This snack is as satisfying as it is easy!

1 slice ham
1 tablespoon cream cheese (to taste, as heavy or thin as you prefer)
1 green onion, cut in half lengthwise

Spread the cream cheese on the ham slice then place the green onion half in the center of the slice. Roll ham around green onion and enjoy.

Dinner

LIME CHICKEN AND RICE

SERVES 2

This dish is hearty and filling, without being too heavy. It's delicious served with green salad and your favorite lime dressing.

1 pound boneless, skinless chicken breast halves
2 cups chicken broth
⅓ cup lime juice
1 clove minced garlic
2 tablespoons butter
½ teaspoon thyme
3 teaspoons lemon juice
2 cups whole rice, cooked
4 green onions, chopped
Salt and pepper to taste
Preheat oven to 350 degrees F

Add all ingredients to a deep dish pan or Dutch overn and cook for 45 minutes or until internal temperature of chicken reaches 165 degrees F

QUINOA MEATLOAF

SERVES 6

Quinoa adds extra protein to this easy, delicious family favorite. For easy servings, this dish is made in a muffin tin. For a great way to add extra calories, serve with a baked potato with butter and toppings. For a leaner version, keep to minimal toppings.

2 pounds ground beef or turkey

1 small onion, chopped

6 ounces tomato paste

2 tablespoons Worcestershire sauce

1 egg, beaten

1 teaspoon salt

1 teaspoon black pepper

¼ cup quinoa

½ cup water

4 tablespoons brown sugar to sprinkle on top

Preheat oven to 350 degrees F. Mix all ingredients, except brown sugar, together in large bowl and divide evenly among the twelve muffin tin cups. Top with brown sugar. Cook for 45 minutes or until internal temperature of meat reaches desired temp (145° F for beef and 165° F for turkey).

BROWN SUGAR SALMON

SERVES 2

Another dish that's so tasty you won't believe how simple it is—just three ingredients! Serve with quinoa and green salad topped with your favorite dressing.

½ cube butter

½ cup brown sugar

2 4-ounce salmon fillets

Preheat oven to 375 degrees F. Place salmon on a large square of aluminum foil. Cut the butter into pieces and place them evenly on the salmon. Sprinkle brown sugar on top wrap the foil.Cook for 25 minutes or until salmon reaches internal temperature of 165 degrees F.

Desserts/Smoothies

ORANGE DREAM SMOOTHIE

SERVES 1

This smoothie is so creamy and sweet, you wouldn't guess there's cabbage and carrots in it!

1 cup vanilla almond milk (you can sub half and half to increase calories)

¾ cup chopped cabbage

1 cup baby carrots, chopped

½ avocado

½ teaspoon orange extract (if you don't have orange, try vanilla)

2½ cups ice cubes

1 orange, peeled

In a blender or food processor, blend all ingredients on high speed until smooth. Enjoy!

POPEYE'S FAVORITE SPINACH SMOOTHIE

SERVES 1

The banana and peanut butter make a delicious creamy shake—and you'll get a dose of one of the world's most nutritious foods, too!

1 cup almond milk (you can sub half and half to increase calories)

½ cup plain Greek yogurt

1 medium banana, frozen

1 tablespoon peanut butter

2½ cups fresh spinach

1 cup ice cubes

In a blender or food processor, blend all ingredients on high speed until smooth. Enjoy!

PROTEIN FRUIT SMOOTHIE

SERVES 1

This smoothie is almost like a fruit and nut parfait, but healthier—it's a great breakfast, snack, or dessert!

> 1 cup frozen berries
> 1 scoop protein supplement
> ½ cup whole milk or your favorite fruit juice
> 1 serving (8 ounces) vanilla Greek yogurt
> 1 teaspoon honey
> Granola

In a blender or food processor, blend all ingredients on high speed until smooth. Top with granola. Enjoy!

CUCUMBER & HONEYDEW SMOOTHIE

SERVES 1

Taste summer in a glass with this fresh, fruity drink.

> 1 medium cucumber peeled and sliced
> 2 cups chopped honeydew melon
> 1 cup passion fruit juice
> 1 scoop vanilla protein
> 1½ cups crushed ice

In a blender or food processor, blend all ingredients on high speed until smooth. Enjoy!

SMOOTHIE ON THE BEACH

SERVES 1

With coconut milk, pineapple, and banana, this smoothie says, Hello, tropical vacation.

1 medium banana, sliced

1 cup baby carrots

1 kiwi, peeled

1 medium apple, peeled and cored

1 cup chopped pineapple

1 orange, peeled

1 cup ice cubes

½ cup coconut milk

In a blender or food processor, blend all ingredients on high speed until smooth. Enjoy!

As you go to the effort to feed your body healthy food, exercise, meditate, and more, you'll find yourself feeling stronger and breathing easier. Another helpful component is to incorporate some stretches that will help you avoid future injury, increase your circulation, improve your breathing, and improve your digestion. I'm talking about yoga. And, yes, you can do it! The next step shows you how.

STEP 9

Try Yoga

You don't have to be great to start, but you have to start to be great.

—ZIG ZIGLAR

By this point, you probably have greater awareness of how essential it is for you to focus more diligently on a few things. Posture, positioning, breathing, and paying attention to your body's signals are a few of the things you need to focus on, not only to get you off to a great start, but to keep you on the path to better health.

One practice that can offer COPD patients many health benefits is yoga. Even if you've never done yoga before, it's easy to get started. Yoga is a discipline originating in ancient India. In the practice of yoga, emphasis is placed upon centering yourself and reducing outside interruptions, allowing you to calm your mind. It heightens your sense of awareness and connectivity, and helps strengthen your mind-body connection. This is very beneficial when you are dealing with physical ailments. You have heard time and again of the direct connection between your emotional state and your physical state. High-stress lifestyles lead to a greater amount of health issues. As you have probably experienced, anxiety perpetuates your shortness of breath. When your physical condition is already compromised, the connection between your mind and your body is more important than ever. And this is where yoga comes in.

Yoga offers many positions that open your chest, strengthen your body, and allow your physical state to improve both immediately as well as over time. On the following pages you will find a few poses you can use that you may find beneficial, especially with practice.

Here are some basic pointers for beginning:

- **Remember to breathe.** While you are performing these positions, remember to breathe. Combining pursed lip breathing (see page 103) with these exercises will help you strengthen your breathing muscles, empty your lungs more completely, and replenish your oxygen supply more efficiently. Keep your oxygen on while performing these exercises. You may need to adjust it to meet your demands, so remember to return it to your resting liter flow upon completion. Make sure you have given your tubing enough slack to allow you to perform these with greater ease.
- Wear loose, comfortable clothing. Bare feet or nonslip socks are fine, too.
- To begin, find a comfortable, firm chair with a sturdy back on it.
- These first exercises are modified from beginning in a standing position; these sitting poses are a good place to start until you are sure your balance and breathing will allow you to complete them without incident. When you are comfortable doing the poses while sitting, you can try them standing.

CHILD'S POSE

Before you begin, it is important to know a restful yoga position called Child's Pose. Child's Pose is used to "reset" when doing yoga. It provides a gentle stretch for the hips, thighs, and ankles. It can also help relieve back pain. Take a moment to rest in Child's Pose anytime you are tired or out of breath, or both. You can stop and rest in Child's Pose whenever you need to during a yoga sequence.

To perform Child's Pose on the floor:

1. Drop your knees to the floor and spread your them wide, big toes touching.
2. Bring your belly to rest between your thighs, and bring your forehead to the floor.

3. From here you can perform two different arm positions. The first is to stretch your arms in front of you, palms facing up. The second is to place your arms next to your sides along your body, palms facing up. You can do whichever is more comfortable for you.

4. If being on the floor is too much for you right now, you can modify Child's Pose for a seated position.

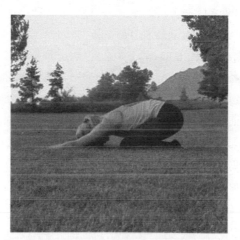

To do Child's Pose in a seated position:

1. Rest leaning forward on the table or another chair in front of you.

2. You can bring your arms up on the table or chair, or you can rest them in your lap or drop them at your sides. This opens up your chest and allows for easier breathing.

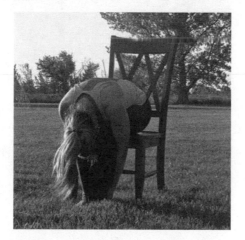

GENTLE SITTING YOGA SEQUENCE

To perform the sequence, follow each pose in order, performing each position three times.

1. CHAIR FORWARD BEND

The first of your poses will begin with a position called Chair Forward Bend.

1. Begin in a seated position sitting square on your buttocks.

2. Lean forward, keeping yourself in a safe position on the chair. Bend from your hips, keeping your back straight, but do not go so far forward that you fall forward.

3. Bring your fingertips in line with your toes and press your palms on the floor or on your legs, if you need to. Engage your quadriceps (muscles in the front of the thighs). This will open up the hamstrings (muscles in the back of the thighs). Bring your weight a little forward.

4. To come out of this pose, slowly raise yourself back to a sitting position. Hold and breathe in through your nose and out through pursed lips for three breaths. Rest and repeat two more times.

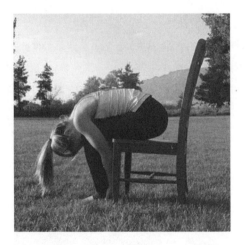

2. CHAIR FISH POSE

This pose is a modified back bend. It serves to open your pectoralis muscles in your chest, the intercostal muscles between your ribs (your accessory breathing muscles), and the upper portion of your hips. Improving the quality of your breathing is a great benefit of this pose. It is also strengthening for the muscles in your back and neck and relieves midback tension. Back bends are known to raise blood pressure, so if you have uncontrolled high blood pressure, you may want to skip this exercise.

1. Normally you would begin by lying on the floor with your knees bent, and feet flat on the floor. For purposes in this book, you will begin in a chair.

2. Bring your arms to your sides, and hold onto the back of your chair. Slide your chest up, arching your back and puffing up your chest.

3. Drop the top of your head back and open your throat.

4. To come out of this pose, slowly bring your head forward and then relax your back against the chair. Hold and breathe in through your nose and out through pursed lips for three breaths. Rest and repeat two more times.

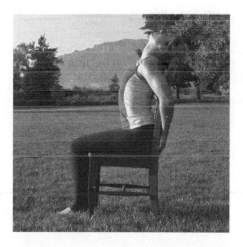

3. CHAIR MOUNTAIN POSE

Mountain Pose improves your posture and strengthens your thighs. It can also help relieve back pain.

To achieve this pose from a chair:

1. Sit up straight with your knees together and your feet aligned forward, big toes touching.

2. Lift up all your toes and let them fan out, and then drop them down forming a sound, solid base. You can separate your heels and ankles if it is uncomfortable. Spread your weight evenly on all corners of the chair.

3. Let your feet and calves root down into the floor. Engage your quadriceps (muscles on the front of your thighs) and draw them upward, causing your kneecaps to rise.

4. Rotate both thighs inward, widening the sit bones, and tuck your tailbone between the sit bones. Pull in your belly slightly.

5. Widen the collar bones: Make sure your shoulders are parallel with your pelvis. Elongate your neck, and raise the top of your head toward the ceiling. Your shoulder blades will slide down your back. This is body alignment. Your hands are brought together in front of you, palms facing each other, fingers extended.

6. Hold and breathe in through your nose, out through pursed lips for three breaths. Rest and repeat.

7. Now drop your arms to your sides and rotate the palms of your hands forward, opening your chest. Hold and breathe in through your nose and out through pursed lips for three breaths. Rest and repeat two more times.

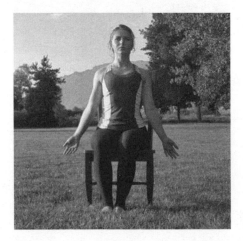

4. CHAIR WARRIOR ONE

1. Sit squarely in your chair, facing forward. Retaining your posture from Mountain Pose, you will raise your arms out to the side and up.

2. Bring your palms together to touch, and gaze upward through your arms toward the thumbs. Your back will arch slightly into a slight back bend. Slide your shoulder blades down the back.

3. Hold and breathe in through your nose and out through pursed lips for three breaths. Rest and repeat.

4. To come out of this pose, return to sitting position and slowly drop your arms to your sides. Rest and repeat two more times.

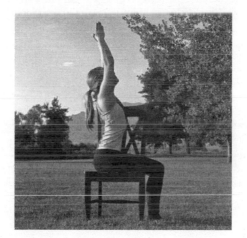

5. CHAIR TRIANGLE POSE

1. Square your hips in your chair and extend your arms to your sides.

2. Bring your left hand to the outside of your right foot or your left arm to the outside of your right leg. This will twist your torso to the right.

3. Bring your arms up to the ceiling, and gaze up through your right fingertips. Try to keep your hips level and parallel to the floor, squarely on the chair. Hold and breathe in through your nose, out through pursed lips for three breaths. Lift back to square position and switch sides, placing your right arm against your left knee and gazing up toward your fingers. Hold and breathe in through your nose and out through pursed lips for three breaths. Lift back to square and rest. Rest and repeat two more times.

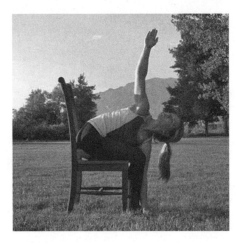

6. CHAIR CAT POSE

1. To perform this stretching exercise, place your hands on your knees. Rest your shoulders and gaze up toward the ceiling.

2. Now arch your back away from you by rounding your spine and pulling your shoulders in. Drop your head and gaze at your navel.

3. Hold and breathe for one breath, in through your nose and out through pursed lips. Rest in normal sitting position and repeat two more times.

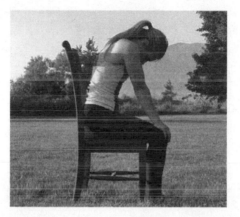

7. CHAIR COBRA POSE

1. To perform Cobra Pose, begin in your sitting position and place your hands on your knees.

2. Slide your chest forward and up, keeping your hands in place.

3. Roll your shoulders back and lift your chest higher, while keeping your ribs lower. Keep your neck neutral. Don't pull or crank it back; rather, leave it in line with your spine.

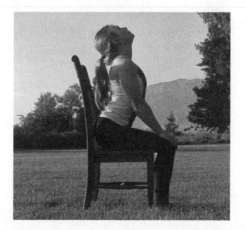

8. CHAIR PIGEON

1. From your sitting position, bring your right ankle to rest on your left knee, keeping the knee in line with your ankle as much as possible.

2. Hold and breathe in through your nose, out through pursed lips for three breaths, resting your hands on your knees. Rest and repeat on the opposite side.

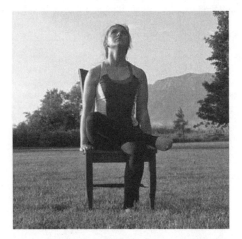

9. CHAIR STRAIGHT LEG EXTENSION

1. Begin in your sitting position. Extend and raise both legs together, straight in front of you.

2. Hold and breathe in through your nose and out through pursed lips for three breaths. Rest and repeat.

3. You may modify this exercise even further by using a yoga strap placed securely under your feet before you lift them and then holding it firmly in both hands while stretching your legs. You may also perform this one leg at a time, if necessary. A yoga strap is made out of cotton or nylon, shaped like a belt, and used to grab bodily limbs you can't reach.

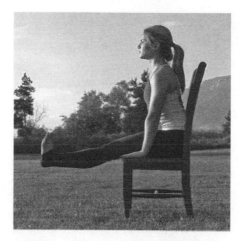

10. CHAIR EAGLE

1. Cross your right thigh over your left thigh. If you can, wrap your right foot around your left calf.

2. Now bring your arms in front of you, and cross the left arm over the right at the elbow.

3. Bend your elbows, and bring your palms together to touch. Lift your elbows slightly from your shoulders away from your ears.

4. Hold and breathe in through your nose and out through pursed lips for three breaths.

5. Straighten your arms and rest. Return your legs to a sitting position. Rest and repeat on the opposite side.

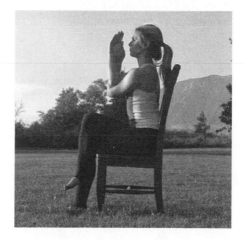

11. CHAIR SPINAL TWIST

For this exercise, turn sideways in your chair. Twist your torso so that your chest faces the back of the chair, and hold on to the chair with your hands. Lengthen your spine upon inhalation and twist on the exhale. Repeat three times, then rest and turn in your chair to the opposite side. Repeat.

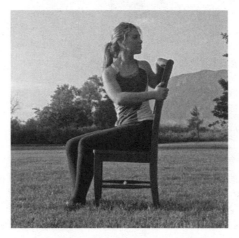

RESTING

After completing this segment of yoga, sit in a comfortable position in your chair, cross your feet, interlace your fingers, and allow yourself to relax and breathe for five minutes. This serves to complete the yoga program you just participated in and allows your brain to correctly process the activities you completed.

Once you have practiced these seated positions and feel you have maximized your benefits here, let yourself advance to a standing version of each position. This will help your progression and offer you new and exciting challenges. You can do these standing next to your chair at first, so it can help stabilize you and provide you with additional confidence until you are ready to try it without the chair.

STANDING YOGA SEQUENCE

To perform the sequence, follow each pose in order.

1. FORWARD BEND

1. Stand with your feet flat on the ground, knees facing forward, toes facing forward, hands to your sides.

2. Bend forward slowly, with your back straight. You want to fold from your hips, deepening your hip creases, instead of from your back.

3. Bring your fingertips in line with your toes, and press your palms flat on the ground. If this is too difficult to do right now, try placing some books or blocks next to your feet and set reaching those as your goal.

4. Engage your quadriceps (muscles in the front of the thighs). This will open up your hamstrings (muscles in the back of the thighs). Bring your weight a little forward.

5. When performing this, you want to keep your weight forward on the balls of your feet and bend your knees slightly in order to keep your palms flat. Then work on straightening your legs.

6. Hold and breathe in through your nose and out through pursed lips for three breaths. Rest and repeat.

7. To come out of this pose, slowly raise yourself back to a standing position.

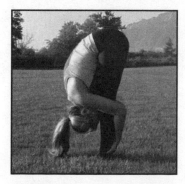

2. FISH POSE

This pose is a back bend. It serves to open your pectoralis muscles in your chest, the intercostal muscles between your ribs (your accessory breathing muscles), and the upper portion of your hips. Improving the quality of your breathing is a great benefit of this pose. It also strengthens the muscles in your back and neck, and relieves midback tension. Back bends are known to raise blood pressure, so if you have uncontrolled high blood pressure, you may want to skip this exercise.

1. Begin by lying on the floor with your knees bent and feet flat on the floor.

2. Bring your arms to your sides, and place your hands so that your thumb can fit underneath your hips.

3. Bend your arms at the elbow, and press into the ground with your forearms. You want your pelvis to rock almost to your sitting bones, accentuating the natural curvature of your lower back.

4. Now slide your chest up and lift your heart to the sky, arching your back where your rib cage is. This elongates your back. Drop the top of your head back and open your throat. You should not feel any discomfort in your lower back.

5. Hold this pose and breathe in through your nose, out through pursed lips for three breaths or up to one minute.

6. To come out of this pose, slowly bring your head forward, tucking your chin and then relax your back against the mat. Rest and repeat.

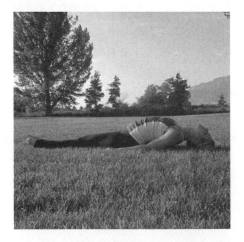

3. MOUNTAIN POSE

Mountain Pose improves your posture and strengthens your thighs. It can also help relieve back pain. To achieve this pose:

1. Stand straight with your knees together and your feet aligned forward, big toes touching.

2. Lift up all your toes and let them fan out, and then drop them down, forming a sound, solid base. You can separate your heels and ankles if it is uncomfortable. Spread your weight evenly on your feet. Let your feet and calves root down into the floor.

3. Engage your quadriceps (muscles on the front of your thighs) and draw them upward, causing your kneecaps to rise.

4. Rotate both thighs inward, widening the sit bones, and tuck your tailbone between the sit bones. Pull your belly in slightly.

5. Widen your collar bones: Make sure your shoulders are parallel with your pelvis. Elongate your neck, and raise the top of your head toward the ceiling. Your shoulder blades will slide down the back. This is body alignment. Your hands are brought together in front of you, palms facing each other, fingers extended.

6. Hold and breathe in through your nose and out through pursed lips for three breaths. Rest and repeat.

7. Now drop your arms to your sides and rotate the palms of your hands forward, opening your chest. Hold and breathe in through your nose and out through pursed lips for three breaths. Rest and repeat.

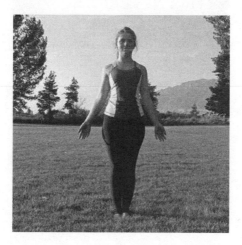

4. WARRIOR ONE

1. When performing Warrior One, you move from Mountain Pose by exhaling as you step your left foot back three or four feet. You want to align your heels one behind the other, and then turn the back foot out by 45 degrees.

2. Turn your hips so that they are both facing directly forward. Keep your back leg straight, and allow your front leg to bend.

3. Inhale as you raise both of your arms from your sides straight over your head, shoulder width apart, palms facing each other. Retaining your posture from Mountain Pose, remember to keep your thighs engaged, your pelvis turned under, and your back straight.

4. Lift your gaze upward through your arms toward the thumbs. Slide your shoulder blades down the back.

5. Hold and breathe in through your nose and out through pursed lips for three breaths or up to one minute. Rest and repeat.

6. To come out of this pose, drop your arms to your sides, placing your hands on your hips. Place the majority of your weight on the forward leg, and bring the backward leg forward. Release yourself into Mountain Pose, take a few deep breaths, and repeat this position on the other side for the same length of time.

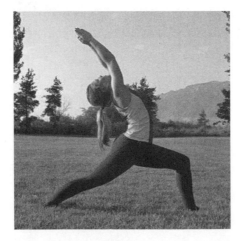

5. TRIANGLE POSE

1. For Triangle Pose, first position yourself in Mountain Pose (standing up straight with your knees together).

2. Take a big step backward, about three feet. Turn your right foot to the side, and keep your left foot facing forward. Your hips are now facing the side of your mat.

3. Inhale, raising your arms to form a "T."

4. Exhale as you bend toward your left foot, bending at your hip and deepening the crease in that joint. Keep your spine long and both sides of your torso of equal length. Allow your dropping arm to float toward your shin. Your top arm is floating up toward the sky, maintaining the "T" shape.

5. Draw in your belly button, gently tuck your chin, and keep your feet firmly planted. Hold and breathe in through your nose and out through pursed lips for three breaths or up to one minute.

6. To exit, gaze toward the bottom leg, and draw up your belly button as you slowly lift back to standing position. Repeat on opposite side from the beginning, and hold for the same amount of time.

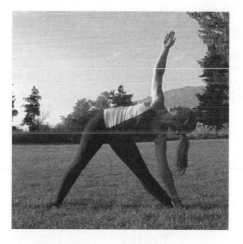

6. CAT POSE

Note: If you suffer from chronic back, neck, wrist, or knee pain, reconsider performing this pose from anything other than the seated position.

1. To perform this stretching exercise, begin on your hands and knees. Place your hands shoulder width apart and your knees hip width apart. Place your hands directly under your shoulders and your knees directly under your hips. Fully spread out your fingers. Place your back into a flat, or horizontal, position with your gaze aimed at the floor beneath you. This is your neutral pose.

2. Tuck your toes underneath your feet to increase the flexibility in your toes. Exhale slowly, raising your belly toward your spine. Lift your spine, rounding it as you tuck your tailbone under and bring your chin toward your chest. Round and raise your back through your breath, pushing yourself up through your shoulders.

3. Rest your shoulders and let the arch in your back rest, your abdominal muscles rest, and the tilt of your hips reverse. Gently turn your gaze up toward the ceiling. Reach your chest away from your waist. Your sit bones will turn upward while your arms remain straight. Watch for your back to sag; you don't want this, and want to remain in a controlled motion.

4. Repeat these movements back and forth several times, feeling the stretch in each vertebra as you increase the mobility of your spine. Be careful not to overextend or create pressure in your spine. Stay within your limits, feeling no pain.

5. To exit, gently return to your neutral pose, untuck your toes, and rest back onto your bent legs, arms outstretched forward in front of you as you rest on your legs in Child's Pose.

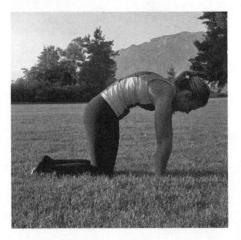

REST IN CHILD'S POSE

1. Drop your knees to the floor and spread your knees wide, big toes touching.

2. Bring your belly to rest between your thighs, and bring your forehead to the floor.

3. From here you can perform two different arm positions. The first is to stretch your arms in front of you, the palms facing up. The second is to place your arms next to your sides along your body, palms facing up. You can do whichever is more comfortable for you.

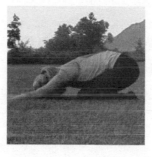

7. COBRA POSE

1. To perform Cobra Pose, gently leave Child's Pose and lie facedown (prone).

2. As you inhale, press your hands into the ground, slowly lifting yourself and lengthening your arms to an almost straightened position, with a small bend in the elbow.

3. Draw your tailbone under, and move your pelvis toward your navel. This pelvic tilt will maintain openness in your lower spine during your arch. Do not rise to the point in which you feel pressure in your lower back.

4. Gently pull your shoulder blades down. Your elbows should be tucked closely to your ribs. Try to recruit your back muscles to work, so your arms are not the only ones benefiting from this pose.

5. Lift your eyes and chin to the point at which you feel your neck open, but not to the point of arching; keep your neck in a neutral position. Breathe in through your nose and out through pursed lips. Hold for three breaths or up to one minute.

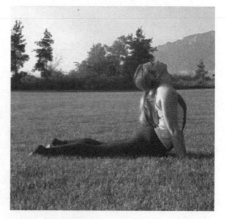

8. PIGEON POSE

1. Sit on the floor and take one knee forward. Take the foot of the bent leg forward to stretch the knee also. Stretch the other leg back, lengthening through the inside of the leg all the way to the big toe.

2. For a little easier pose, place the hands on the mat in front of your bent leg, or place your hands under your hips for a slightly harder pose. If you place your finger tips on the mat you will also get a better stretch around your shoulders.

3. Hold and breathe in through your nose and out through pursed lips for three breaths. Rest and repeat on opposite side.

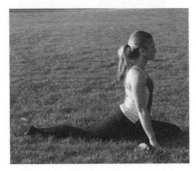

9. STRAIGHT LEG EXTENSION

1. Sit on the floor.

2. Extend and raise both legs together, straight in front of you. Hold and breathe in through your nose and out through pursed lips for three breaths. Rest and repeat.

3. You may modify this exercise even further by using a yoga belt placed securely under your feet before you lift them and hold it firmly in both hands while stretching your legs. You may also perform this one leg at a time, if necessary.

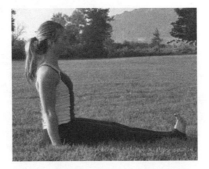

10. EAGLE POSE

1. Standing Eagle is performed by standing on one foot (we will start on the left), crossing your right thigh over your left thigh, and wrapping your right foot around the calf of your left leg.

2. Now bring your arms in front of you and cross them, the left arm over the right at the elbow. Bend your elbows and bring your palms to touch. Lift your elbows slightly from your shoulders away from your ears.

3. Hold and breathe in through your nose and out through pursed lips for three breaths. Straighten your arms and rest. Unwind your legs and return to standing position, feet shoulder width apart, toes facing forward.

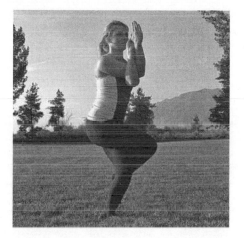

11. SPINAL TWIST

1. Sit on the floor, stretching your legs out in front of you. Bend your knees, placing your feet on the floor. Now slide your left foot under your right leg so it is toward the outside of your right hip. Lay the outside of your left leg on the floor and place your right foot over your left leg with the bottom of your foot on the floor as if you are standing. Your right knee will stand up toward the ceiling.

2. Exhale and twist your body toward the inside of your right thigh. Press your right hand on the floor behind your right buttock and rest your left upper arm on the outside of your right thigh near your knee. Pull your front torso and inner right thigh together.

3. Sit up straight to lengthen the back through your tailbone and lean backward just slightly.

4. Twist your torso by turning to the right.

5. Turn your head toward the right following your twist, or turn it to the left to counteract the twist.

6. Breathe in while lifting through your sternum, twisting a little more with each exhalation, holding for 30 seconds, and let go upon exhalation. Repeat on the opposite side.

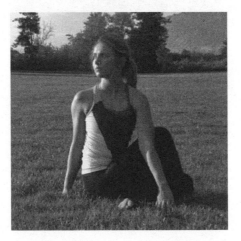

You may be hesitant as you start out. Remember to go slow, and always pay attention to your breathing. Also remember that this isn't a race: Yoga is about slow movements, done with focus and intention. Hopefully, you'll fall in love with it, and you'll reap the many benefits. As you learn your yoga program and work it successfully, you will begin to recognize your mind-body connection and even learn to nurture it. That is great and very important! But as important as it is, it is not the only relationship that is important for you to foster. What about the other people in your life? The next step talks about maintaining important connections, especially when times are tough.

Stay Connected

Thankfully, persistence is a great substitute for talent.

—STEVE MARTIN

As your disease progresses, you may find that your role with some of the people in your life changes. Where you once may have been a caregiver, you are becoming the receiver. For many this is a difficult transition, especially in the beginning.

Lots of people struggle with letting their children, friends, or family become their caretakers. You may be used to providing for your family, being the strong arm that was needed so often, and being the emotional protector of the relationship and those you love. Maybe you used to be responsible for caring for your family's daily physical needs, such as providing meals and a clean, welcoming home. Living with COPD may mean that now others need to help you move things around the house, drive you places, do chores for you, cook for you, and more. You will inevitably have times when you feel angry at your inability to perform activities you used to so easily do. Many times it is simply directed at your disease, itself. Be careful to keep communication lines open so misdirected anger doesn't hurt those you love.

It can be an unsatisfying bridge to cross, and can leave both men and women struggling with painful feelings of uselessness and isolation. But the good news is you can find effective ways to cope that will reestablish your sense of well-being and make this transition a smoother one. It's all about maintaining your relationships and friendships, communicating, and staying connected to others.

Let's take a look at Pat. When Pat first came into therapy, one of the primary concerns shared with me by her husband was that she just wasn't herself anymore. She wasn't eating right, she wasn't happy anymore. She had gone from being the center of life for her family to being the center of concern for those who loved her. She still found the most joy in her grandchildren and spoke of them often, but the light that was once in her eyes had diminished so much that her husband stood there in front of me in tears, begging for help.

"Please, help me find my wife. I know she's in there," was his plea.

I put myself to work. Each session she came in for therapy I tried to focus with her on the emotional and mental side of the disease, working side by side with her during her exercise routine. In our education sessions, I was sure to ask her questions to help her become more engaged and involved. After a few weeks, the results were coming in fast and were easily defined. Her appetite improved. She smiled more. She began participating in more things at home. She reconnected with her husband in ways they both thought were never to be experienced again. She was alive.

So, how did this disease affect her relationships? If she had not chosen to be actively involved in her care and had the opportunity of finding the necessary tools not been presented to her, she very well may have continued down the same road I found her on. It had distanced her from her most intimate relationships—her children, her friends, her husband—as she prepared to die instead of choosing to live. Is she entitled to bad days? Sure, she is! But the key was to fight, to not succumb to that way of thinking chronically. The next time her husband came to me he was, again, in tears, only this time they were tears of joy, tears of gratitude, and tears of a whole heart instead of a broken one. He hugged me and cried, saying, "I have my wife back. Thank you." And then left, smiling and wiping tears from his cheeks as he waved back to me. I also wiped tears from my own cheek as I waved back.

INTIMACY, NOT ISOLATION

When we talk about intimacy, it relates to various aspects of our lives in several ways. Intimacy is having a close familiarity or friendship and is a quality of many of our most important relationships. How does living with a chronic disease affect intimacy in your life?

Chronic disease can take its toll on relationships if it isn't discussed, which can lead to feelings of isolation, distance, and loneliness. This can have a drastic impact on the level of intimacy experienced in all relationships, which delivers a strong blow to all those involved. But it doesn't have to be that way. A little discussion and conversation mixed with understanding and love can greatly improve the situation. This isn't to say that *all* conversation, or even a majority of the conversation surrounding you, needs to be about your disease or condition. That can also become a problem, but finding a middle ground that opens the doors for questions and removes difficult barriers will provide the best result. This degree of conversation will be different for each individual, couple, family, and group of friends, but it can be found, and for the wellness of all involved it needs to be.

Intimacy comes in many forms. Touch, a hug, even the look in an eye can have an intimate feeling attached to it. These release endorphins into our blood, which affect us physically. Just as your deep-breathing exercises will have a physical effect on the cellular level, human touch and intimacy have a similar effect. The biological need we, as humans, have to be touched and loved is indisputable. Studies show that human beings need nine points of contact per day to function optimally. Consider this when you need that connection to take place. Touch is a biological need that is essential for our emotional health.

Studies have been done on children that have not had healthy, loving touch from caretakers or loved ones compared to children that have been given an abundance of attention. The emotional development and well-being of those who are touched and cared for appropriately far exceed the emotional development and well-being of those who do not. We need touch. We need love. We also need to love others. If our emotions so strongly affect our physical well-being, doesn't it make sense to ensure the continuation of the healthy relationships in your life?

STAYING CONNECTED WITH YOUR FAMILY AND FRIENDS

What and how can things change and leave you feeling whole? It could be that you now share your secrets of how to fix that oil leak with your grandson, advising him how to do it and supervising his work. You may direct others on how to make your famous Thanksgiving dinner instead of cooking it for them. You may teach your daughter how to clean things and instruct her while she scrubs your house, instead of doing it yourself, and you may offer direction on what way you would like the garage cleaned out or the trees planted instead of doing them yourself. It's simply realigning yourself to your new normal, letting people serve you (as you taught them to do through your years of service to them), and graciously accepting their service because they enjoy doing it, they love you, and they grow in the process. You wouldn't want to interrupt that, would you?

Try to realize that while your roles may have changed, your value has not because your value is not placed on the things you do. Your family still needs you, you still matter, and your place in the family is still as important as it has ever been. Remember all those wonderful, caring things you did for your children and family, your friends, and your neighbors? Well, now it is their turn to show you how much they appreciate what you have done and return the love and support you have given to them over the years.

If you are on oxygen, at some point in time you will need to introduce your family and friends to it. There's an idea of how to do that below. If there are smaller children around, this is a good opportunity to let them touch it, feel it, and listen to it. This will remove some of the curiosity they have and help alleviate any fear or apprehension they may have in dealing with it. Explain what it is, what it does, how it works, and how it helps you. Help them understand why you need it by giving them a straw to breathe through and having them jump up and down or run in place. This offers perspective to them. You could even let them try it on—you can also purchase an extra hose for them to try on instead of using yours. In fact, you can do the same with your CPAP/BiPAP mask. Let them hold it to their face. Turn it into a game. That way, when they see it on you, they will not be afraid and will be more accepting and less concerned about it.

Another trick you can try is to exercise with your family. Teach them your breathing exercises and ask them to do your yoga with you. This will help them become familiar with your routine and what you can tolerate. One exercise, mentioned in other areas of this book, which helps strengthen your breathing muscles is playing the harmonica. Singing together is great, too. These are both activities you can participate in with a group, be it friends or family. It will do them as much good as it does you! All of these ideas will help them understand you better and understand your disease more fully. This will reduce your anxiety and theirs, which is important, because when your anxiety level decreases, your breathing ability improves!

Going to church or otherwise participating in whatever faith you may be a part of is also something to take into consideration. In many church organizations volunteering for various callings and/or positions is a vital part of a successful organization. For many people this is tremendously important for both their spiritual well-being as well as their sense of self and declaration of who they are. Many people place a higher amount of concern on fulfilling these callings than other areas of their lives, which is evidence of the importance of their faith. While that faith may be in large part what helps them carry on through difficult times such as when dealing with a chronic disease, it is also important to realize that your ability to perform tasks in this aspect may, at some point, also be affected. The important thing to remember is that, once again, you are not valued on what you give, you are valued simply by being you. That being said, in most organizations there are ways to volunteer and "give back" that do not require a great amount of physical exertion, if that becomes difficult for you. There are many things, such as contributing to newsletters, being in leadership positions in which you can teach and delegate, teaching itself (if that much talking isn't too difficult to do), and office/clerical work that needs to be done. The point being that when serving is needed, you can still serve in ways that can be adjusted to your ability to do so in a healthy manner. Don't risk your health to do things that are out of your safety zone.

Here are a few more tips for maintaining friendships:

- Don't put energy into trying to evaluate others motives and focus instead on what they can do to support you.
- Remember this is YOUR life, and you can turn what is in your control into what you want and need.
- Give yourself what you need instead of waiting for someone else to give it to you. You know what you need, take the time to give it to yourself.
- If you'd really rather do something yourself, or do it your way, thank the person who offers help . . . and ask whether he or she might be available to assist you in another way.
- Maintain friendships through e-mail, phone calls, and social media.
- Seek out friends and acquaintances who understand how you feel and/ or suffer from a similar or the same situation.

STAYING CONNECTED AT THE OFFICE

What about your colleagues? Changes at work can also be difficult to navigate. It often means dealing with lost work days, management of symptoms and recovery time, and needing to work around medical or rehab appointments. For some, chronic disease may mean adjusting or changing duties within the same company, but for some it could mean early retirement, loss of employment, finding new employment, or retraining for a new career altogether. Some suggestions to coping with changes at the office include:

- Keep a clear line of communication.
- Be up front with your co-workers about your condition—as you feel comfortable discussing.
- Check your employer's sick and disability policies.
- Talk with your HR manager.
- If your current duties require active physical labor, discuss with your doctor and manager how to approach a modified work schedule.
- Become familiar, if you're not already, with your health insurance policy and what items are covered or not covered.
- Check into your HSA, if you have one, and budget for future needs.
- Revisit your benefits during your company's open enrollment period and reevaluate your plan to make sure you have the best coverage for yourself and your situation.
- Look into long- and short-term disability insurance and become familiar with how and when to use those.
- Become familiar with purchasing a COBRA plan or maintaining your own insurance plan if your ability to continue working is challenged.

WHAT TO SAY

Sometimes your COPD can feel like the elephant in the room. Depending on the relationships you have, and who you are speaking with, what you share about your health will be different. Your adult children may know better than a colleague about your condition and your unique way of processing things. A close friend may be the one you share difficulties with and may be the one you talk with the most, and those conversations will be different than what you may discuss with a neighbor.

You are the one that gets to decide how much each person with whom you are in relationship learns about your condition and difficulties, but remember, you are working toward accepting your COPD for what it is and it is nothing to be embarrassed about or ashamed of.

So, let's review a few statements or conversation starters you can practice and use when dealing with different people. The following statements and practices were tried out by patients while writing this book. They have all been used successfully many times and helped those involved establish ways of communicating their condition at any given time and in regard to the many facets of their illness with various people and the many differing relationships they have.

A surprisingly easy topic to begin with is oxygen. If you wear oxygen, use that as a conversation starter. Some people have a harder time than others when it comes to needing oxygen. The tubing on their face bothers some more than others, the tube is more annoying to some than it is to others, and the attention it brings to the tube wearer is more difficult for some than for others. You can always say something like, "How do you like my oxygen?" followed by, "I can still do most things; this stuff here just helps keep me going!" Some people, in a joking manner, call their oxygen tubing their "chain" and refer to their tanks or concentrator as their "anchor," a new "ball and chain," or "my new best friend." Your casual acknowledgment of the tubing may relieve others of the discomfort of not knowing whether it is okay to express their concern or curiosity about your health. In addition, opening the conversation yourself will allow you to steer it in a positive direction. It is a way of letting people know you do have a breathing issue, yet in a manner that also tells them it isn't getting you down.

One of the things that can be difficult is needing recovery time during outings. Many people feel embarrassed that they need to sit down in a store or rest on a shopping cart. There are more hints on how to do this in the section about positioning (see page 107), but simply smiling and looking confident while you are recovering, catching your breath, or just resting can help relieve attention from those around you. You can try doing something like feigning reading a book, or say something such as a simple "Hello" and smile to those who walk by. If they stop and talk, they will most likely ask you if you need or want anything. To this you can simply reply, "Just resting my feet, thanks." Or "I'm just waiting for someone." If you are too breathless to speak, you can simply smile and shake your head with a grateful wave of your hand. Most people will respect this response.

Other Helpful Conversation Starters

In regard to altering the way you do things:

"I have found that if I do things this way, it works better for me."

"I'm switching things up a bit this time."

"Let's try to do this instead, as something new."

"The older I get, the wiser I get. I found a better way of doing that!"

In regard to mealtime:

"I've decided to stop rushing through meals the way I used to."

"I've discovered that when I eat more slowly, I really taste and enjoy my food."

"More frequent, smaller meals seem to agree with me better than eating a few large ones. Have you tried it?"

"Extra calories are actually good for me these days: If I want some ice cream, I eat it."

In regard to needing to rest:

"Let's look at the scenery for a minute."

"Would you like to sit down and people-watch with me? It's fascinating!"

"How about we take a breather for a minute?"

"Let's let these people behind us pass; they seem to be in much more of a hurry than we are."

"Would you like to stop for a minute to get something to drink? I'd love some cold water."

SEXUAL INTIMACY WITH YOUR PARTNER

Just because you have COPD doesn't mean sexual intimacy can't still be an important part of your life. Some people seldom have sexual problems in relation to their lung disease, whereas others have more frequent and more persistent issues. It is healthy and normal for you to have questions. You might wonder about things like, "Will my oxygen limit me?" "Is it safe to have sex?" "What can I do when I feel short of breath?" "Do people in my condition participate in that activity?" Or "What is the best way for us to be intimate?" Again, it is healthy and normal to ask these questions, and even better, it is healthy and normal to have them answered. A loving relationship with your partner will help you overcome these issues and the accompanying emotions that are affecting both of you.

Although it may be difficult, communication is a great place to start. It may be helpful to make a list of your concerns. Use your journal to compile a list of your concerns and also some thoughts about what you think your partner may be feeling. Your partner may have concerns regarding your health and safety. You may have questions about your ability to participate, especially if you have struggled in the past. As with every other part of your life, this may require making some adjustments. Set aside a time to talk that will leave you free of distractions (such as television, children, or telephones).

When you are talking together, be specific about things that make it difficult for you both, as well as things that enhance the experience together. Again, it might be easiest if you think about these things beforehand and write them down. Aside from dealing with the lung disease, you may also be coping with physical changes that happen with age. Consider these things, and don't hesitate to talk with your doctor or nursing staff.

If you are a woman, you may find you need additional lubrication. If this is the case, speak with your provider about the possibility of needing hormone replacement therapy or creams, and don't hesitate to use a lubricant. If you do, make sure it is a water-soluble lubricant and not one that is petroleum based. A lubricant can help reduce irritation or avoid irritation and make things more comfortable for you.

As a man, you may find you need help achieving a desired erection. Again, don't be afraid to speak to your provider about medications or methods you can use to help you with the ability to perform, increase your stamina, or have the ability to participate in sexual intimacy.

EXERCISE AND YOUR SEX LIFE

Most people are aware that exercise is proven to improve physical condition, mental alertness, and self-esteem. What you might not know is that it can also be beneficial to your sex life. During sex (just like during exercise), most people experience an increase in respirations and heart rate. In fact, the amount of energy required during sex could be compared to a brisk walk or climbing stairs.

You have been learning how to breathe efficiently and effectively during activities of your daily life, and hopefully you have been practicing them. (It is never a good idea to try to learn those patterns when you are feeling panicked or struggling.) Because sex requires a higher level of activity than normal, everyday actions, it is important to apply the rules of the ABCDEs of COPD to this activity as you will many others. Yes, it may seem like a lot of planning, but this is just a part of your new normal—and it will help you and your partner enjoy being physically intimate without worries of an exacerbation or other problem.

First, take **aim**. If possible, plan sex for the time of day when you feel your best. This may vary from your traditional schedule or timing, but that is all right. A lot of things are changing, and this is just another one of those things. Many people feel their best in late morning or early afternoon.

It is also a good idea to plan this activity, as well as all activities, around your medications. If you take a bronchodilator, talk to your doctor about planning around it. Also, keep your emergency inhaler close by in case you need it. It will allow you to breathe easier, thus reducing panic and assisting you in feeling more relaxed.

Try to wait two to three hours after a large meal. A full stomach increases your shortness of breath, which could make sexual activity difficult. Decide what time of day is best and talk with your partner. Chances are he or she will be willing to help you any way possible. And remember, if you would put oxygen on to go for a walk or climb stairs, put it on now. Ensure that you have turned it up to the proper level for activity. (Try wrapping the tubing around the back of your head and tightening it up there. Remember to improvise if you need to.)

Second, **get your bearings**. Increase your activity level slowly. Remember to use your breathing exercises if you begin to feel short of breath. Try not to hold your breath. Instead, breathe fully through all stages of your sexual experience. Orgasm has proven benefits both emotionally and physically, decreasing stress, improving blood flow, improving health and overall well-being, and improving or maintaining a healthy relationship, but if you can't relax, it will be much harder to attain. Pace yourself, focus on relaxing and feeling everything during your experience. Focus on your partner, as he or she focuses on you. Take your time; don't rush. Get comfortable and enjoy yourself.

Third, **calculate**. Calculate the benefits and risks of participating in sexual activity right now. Are you having a good day? Are you healthy today? Are your meds working correctly? Add up your pros and cons, and if your numbers add up, make pleasuring each other your priority. Relax and allow yourself this time. Breathe.

Fourth, **decide and be deliberate**. Try something *new*, if you need to. Modifications to what you used to do has worked on many other things; apply it deliberately to this area of your life, as well. Try a less strenuous position. If there are positions that increase coughing, or make it more difficult to breathe, avoid them. Positions that require you to use your arms and upper body strength will tend to be more strenuous and are positions you should think about avoiding. Use additional pillows for support, if necessary. Try to avoid positions that restrict your lungs.

Let the partner without the breathing difficulties do most of the moving and don't be afraid to change positions often, if you need to. Keeping it rhythmic will help your breathing. Most of all, remember that these are pointers to help get you started, not limit you. You can and should do what works for you. Remember to keep your partner included in your feelings. Remember to keep his or her feelings in mind. This is new to your partner, as well.

Next, conserve your **energy**. In my experience in talking through this with most of my patients and many others, it seems to be a commonality that moving too quickly or neglecting to conserve energy previously in the day for this activity can put quite a damper on the experience. John, a recent patient, stated how much he missed making love to his wife. By reviewing their schedules and other activities, he found that he could easily conserve enough energy throughout the day to participate in this activity that they so missed. After talking it through (one of the most important things you can do as a couple), he and his wife discovered they simply had to make a few adjustments that truly had a substantial payout!

Most of all, remember that time together is important. Being physically close to your partner results in loving feelings and brings you closer together. The communication process your changes are requiring may very well bring you closer together, as well. Relying on each other and trusting in one another will result in more fulfillments in your relationship. Having chronic lung disease does not mean your life has to end. It does not have to interfere with satisfaction. Your health-care providers (doctors, nurses, respiratory therapists, and psychological counselors) are here to help you. Use your resources, ask questions, and talk to you partner. Your sexuality is an important part of your relationship and your life.

TAKE CHARGE OF YOUR LIFE

Here are a few pointers to help you feel more positive, help overcome the depression and emotional struggles you may be facing, and feel better overall. Don't forget, if left unattended, chronic illness can really take a toll on you, greatly reduce your quality of life, and change the quality of intimacy in your relationships. Using some simple tools and following a few rules will help you stay on top of it all. You can live life to its fullest within your limits, maintain a healthy level of intimacy, and gain the value we all need from healthy relationships.

Find new meaning, new purpose to your life. Practice gratitude daily. Let your family and friends help you. Make a list of the things you are grateful for and read them aloud each morning and anytime during the day when you are feeling down. One of the worst habits of chronically unhappy people is that they tend to focus on the negative things in both their lives and the world. Have you ever just said, "Thank you [to what or whoever your higher power is or just to the universe] for waking me up today"? That statement in itself carries great strength and helps put things in perspective. Sometimes we have to do that several times during the day, other times, once is enough to make a difference. Listen to your needs, and don't be afraid to tend to them.

Give yourself and let others around you give you, permission to slow down. It's okay to do things differently. Your body will thank you, your soul will thank you, and those who love you will thank you. It is permissible to shift gears from the pace you once ran your life at, establish your new pace, which may even vary from day to day, and your relationships will benefit from your decision to do this.

Speaking of relationships, surround yourself with loving, helpful people. They want to help you; you need to let them do this. You will soon find that you will all feel better.

When talking to your support system, be honest. When talking to yourself, be honest. Honesty will help relieve stress and help you focus more clearly on what your body needs right now.

Find the "now." Find it and settle in. Live in it every day. Absorb the goodness of each day and let the bad moments coexist with them without dwelling on those.

EPILOGUE: YOUR SUCCESS STARTS TODAY

The best way to predict your future is to create it.

—ABRAHAM LINCOLN

Now that you understand what is happening in your lungs, are more familiar with some of the topics that are now a part of your daily life, and have the tools to organize the elements of your health care and lung disease, it is time to put them to use. Following this program enables you to consistently be on top of your game. When you listen to your body and are well engaged in your care, you're able to reverse the COPD Downward Spiral and actively take charge of your health.

You'll also want to be sure to fill out the charts in the Appendix (pages 285–307) so that you can stay well organized and present any information to your health-care providers anytime you need to. Remember, you are your own best advocate. My hope is that with the COPD Solution, you have a clearer understanding of what lies ahead and are already practicing the behaviors and life skills to face both your trials and your successes head on.

If you've been following each step of this program as you've made your way through the book, congratulations! No doubt you've already experienced some positive changes. Let's take a look at how far you've come!

PART 1: LIVING WITH CHRONIC LUNG DISEASE

- You know which conditions you have that make up your COPD.
- You know your symptoms.
- You have learned the Borg Scale, so you can rate your level of difficulty in accomplishing tasks.
- You also have learned that pacing yourself will present you with definite rewards of fewer recovery days.

- You understand your PFTs and other tests that are done to not only diagnosis your lung disease but also monitor it.
- With this understanding, you will have the ability to perform your tests with less anxiety and a clear understanding of what your expectations as a patient are.
- You understand what each measurement represents, knowing that if you forget any particular part all you have to do is thumb back to a specific page and you have all the information you need at your fingertips.

PART 2: THE COPD SOLUTION PROGRAM

Step 1: Make Peace with COPD
- You've accepted your diagnosis of COPD.
- You have worked through the stages of grief often associated with loss.

Step 2: Start Oxygen Therapy
- Your oxygen is no longer a mystery. You now understand how it is helping you breathe and understand why you have it and why you need it. Gaining knowledge of the various delivery and storage systems helps you find the system that works best for you.
- You have your oxygen and DME equipment provider listed on your tracking sheet.
- You have listed the specific numbers and information for each device you use.
- Your "Oxygen in Use" signs are hanging in the appropriate locations so that emergency personnel and visitors are well aware.
- Your "No Smoking" sign is hanging up, and your friends and family members understand the urgency of this situation. They support you in it. This relieves some of your apprehensions about using your oxygen, and you now realize that it is a necessary part of your life, and realize the gift of life it gives you.

Step 3: Breathe Easier
- You know how to use pursed lip breathing and other breathing techniques.
- Remember, smell the cake, blow out the candles.
- Belly breathing is important, too! Breathe all the way down into your belly and release through pursed lips.

Step 4: Conserve Your Energy
Making lifestyle adjustments to conserve energy will prove to be one of the most effective choices you make.

- You know the ABCDE tips for energy conservation. Find your own, share them with others, and use them often. This is not lazy! It is smart, useful, and necessary.
- You've planned your hours, days, and weeks to organize your activities most effectively. Prioritizing will help you plan.
- You now pace yourself. This is of utmost importance and must become second nature.
- You listen to your body, not your to-do list.
- You use positioning to help you focus and use your breathing exercises and relaxation to help relieve the episodes of shortness of breath. Find the positions that work best for you and practice them often, prior to the occurrence of an urgent situation.
- You practice your positive self statements to help you prepare for difficult and emotionally charged situations. The power of positive thinking on our health has been proven many times over in scientific studies done all over the world. Your mind and body can work as one to strengthen you or to weaken you. It is up to you to decide which it will be every day.

Step 5: Prevent Flare Ups: Use Your Meds Effectively

It is time to celebrate because your medications are no longer a mystery or overwhelming!

- You know the order in which to use your medications.
- Your new understanding of how to properly use your inhaler or nebulizer (including cleaning it) has given your medications the opportunity to work their best.
- You know how and when to increase your rescue breather. Using your rescue inhaler is more of a planned and purposeful thing now, and you understand that the use of this is a great tool, not only in helping you breathe better, but in monitoring the effectiveness of your maintenance medications.
- Because you are more familiar with your breathing patterns and behavior, you know how to watch for exacerbations.
- You know how to track your symptoms.
- You know how to track your medications, and have been given the tools to do so, which will enable you to be well prepared at each of your appointments and in case of emergency.
- You are learning what your triggers are, and tracking them to watch for exacerbations. This will help you avoid those triggers, which will improve your likelihood of a greater number of "good breathing days."

- You are rinsing your mouth and doing what you need to do to avoid thrush.
- You have a greater understanding of when to contact your physician if an increase of medication is necessary.
- You know what a valuable tool your pharmacist is in assisting you with anything regarding your medications.
- Your refills are marked on your calendar, both the order date and the pickup date. If your meds are mailed, your expectant date of arrival is noted on your calendar. These dates ensure that you will not go for any amount of time without your breather medications.

Step 6: Go to Pulmonary Rehab
- You've found an effective pulmonary rehabilitation program in your area.
- You've learned new things about your body and stretching your limits. Remember . . . it is with stretching that we grow. It is with growing that we progress. It is with progression that we succeed.
- You've take your exercise home with you. Once you are discharged from PR, ensure your continued well-being by utilizing the home exercise program your therapist designs for you. This will continue to benefit you every single day.

Step 7: Quit Smoking
- If you have quit smoking, take a moment to congratulate yourself!
- If you have not quit yet, take a moment when you can and reread this step on page 187.
- You've broken down your goal into steps and are rewarding yourself for progress.
- Check with your local health department and state health agencies. They will have additional resources for you to use, if you would like.
- You know the mode of quitting is a little different for everyone. The mode is not important. You do what works best for you. The important thing is to quit. You deserve to be smoke free. You can do it!

Step 8. Choose Foods for Better Breathing
- You have reevaluated your nutritional habits. Remember, your prescribed medications are not your only medications. Food is medicine. It can help or hinder, depending on what we choose to use it for.
- You have gained knowledge that will help you move better, breathe better, and live better.

- You've cut down on refined sugars, carbonated beverages, saturated fat, trans fat, and salt.
- Your anxiety regarding food and eating has eased as you practice pacing your breathing with your eating.
- You're breaking the COPD Cycle of Malnutrition. Your diet will help you avoid the effects of malnutrition and help you gain the elements of nutrition you need. You will be so successful at this.

Step 9: Try Yoga
- You've started practicing yoga and relax regularly.
- You've strengthened your mind-body connection.
- You've improved your breathing muscles and your ability to use them.

Step 10: Stay Connected
- You've committed to staying connected with family and friends, using conversation starters when things get difficult.
- You and your partner have used the ABCDEs of COPD to help increase intimacy and have a joyful sex life.
- You're taking steps to help you feel more positive, help overcome the depression and emotional struggles you may be facing, and feel better overall.

Reviewing and practicing the points on your checklists, referring back to the text when needed, as well as completing and filling out your action plans and charts will make you a disease managing pro! You will have the organization, the skill, the tools, and the know-how to manage your disease effectively. You will even be able to share your knowledge with others you may know or meet that are struggling just like you were! Now, there's a payday that makes it all worthwhile! Did you ever think, before you started this program, that you would be so capable? Well, I did. I've seen it happen time and time again. Many patients start working this program in what they feel are their own personal pits of despair and come out on the other end smiling, moving, traveling, living, and loving, even teaching others how to live. These are my own, favorite, personal paydays. I can't tell you how many tears of joy have been shed each time a patient hits a personal milestone. You are going to do so well! I can't wait to hear about it!

You are becoming very strong and capable! Having this understanding helps you take care of yourself so you can stop the progression of COPD in its tracks. Your awareness of your own body and its needs is heightened through the knowledge you are gaining. You will even find yourself becoming an advocate with those you meet, educating and sharing the knowledge you are continually gaining with them and helping them through struggles you are already familiar with.

Pat yourself on the back for taking a proactive approach in dealing with the issues you are facing. Pat yourself on the back for taking care of yourself. Pat yourself on the back for the way your activity levels will increase and the progression of your lung disease will slow. You deserve it. You are welcoming the acceptance of your disease, but not succumbing to it. And remember,

> *You are braver than you believe, stronger than you seem, and smarter than you think.*
>
> —WINNIE THE POOH
> (MY FAVORITE YELLOW BEAR)

GLOSSARY

Accessory muscles: The intercostal muscles that surround the rib cage. It is used as a secondary muscle group in situations involving compromised ventilation such as chronic lung disease.

Airway: The passageway by which air passes from the nose or mouth into the air sacs of the lungs.

Alveoli: The air cells, or air sacs, of the lung, formed by the terminal dilation of tiny air passageways.

Antibiotic: Any of a large group of chemical substances used chiefly in the treatment of infectious diseases.

Anti-inflammatory: A medication used to reduce inflammation either locally or systemically.

Antioxidant: An enzyme that is capable of counteracting the damaging effects of oxidation in animal tissue.

Asthma: A disorder of the respiratory system characterized by bronchospasm, wheezing, and difficult expirations. It is often accompanied by coughing and a feeling of constriction in the chest.

Beta-agonist: A group of medications that primarily affect the muscles surrounding the airways in the lungs, causing the muscles to relax and widening the airways as a result.

BiPAP: Bilevel positive airway pressure treatment used for sleep apnea.

Bronchiectasis: A disease in which the bronchial tubes are distended, causing secretions to pool in airways.

Bronchodilator: A substance that causes dilation of constricted bronchial tubes to aid in breathing.

Calorie: Term used to express the heat output of an organism and the fuel or energy value of food.

Capillaries: A minute blood vessel between the terminations of the arteries and the beginning of the veins.

Carbohydrate: Compounds of carbon, hydrogen, and oxygen (as sugars, starches, and celluloses), most of which are formed by green plants and which constitute a major class of food.

Carbon dioxide (CO2): A colorless, odorless, incombustible gas present in the atmosphere and formed during chemicals breaking down in the body and released during respiration.

Chronic bronchitis: A condition of bronchitis persisting for two or more consecutive months of two or more consecutive years.

COPD (chronic obstructive pulmonary disease): Consisting of any two of the following three diseases: asthma, emphysema, or chronic bronchitis.

CPAP (continuous positive airway pressure): A treatment used to hold airways open as treatment for sleep apnea.

Cystic fibrosis (CF): A hereditary, chronic disease of the exocrine glands characterized by the production of viscid mucus that obstructs pancreatic ducts and bronchial tubes leading to infection and fibrosis.

Deconditioning: A condition in which there is a reduced functional capacity of the body due to chronic illness.

Deoxygenated: A condition of having oxygen removed from something.

Depression: A condition of general emotional withdrawal; sadness greater and more prolonged than that warranted by any objective reason.

Diaphragm: A muscular wall separating the thoracic cavity from the abdominal cavity.

Diaphragmatic breathing: Breathing method focused on using intentional distention of the diaphragm to use the lower lobes of the lungs.

DPI (dry powder inhaler): A type of inhaler that contains a dry powder as opposed to a mist. To be taken by those who have a strong inhalation ability, with fast, deep breath.

Emphysema: A chronic, irreversible lung disease characterized by enlargement of and accompanied by destruction of the tissue lining the alveolar walls.

Fat: Any of several greasy substances forming the chief part of adipose (fat) tissue of animals. Also present in plants.

Fiber: Also called bulk, dietary fiber, roughage; the structural part of plant products that consists of carbohydrates, that are wholly or partially indigestible, and when eaten stimulate peristalsis in the intestine.

Food Guide Pyramid: A model after which to fashion your nutrition, a nutritional guideline.

Inhaler: A device used for the delivery of inhaled medications.

Intranasal: Within the nasal cavity.

Isometric exercise: Exercises to strengthen specific muscles or shape the figure by pitting one muscle part against another or against an immovable object in a strong but motionless action, as by pressing the fist of one hand against the palm of the other.

Isotonic exercise: Exercise to increase strength, power, and endurance based on lifting a constant amount of weight at variable speeds through a range of motion.

Macronutrient: Any nutritional component of a diet that is required in large amounts.

Malnutrition: Improper or lack of balanced nutrition.

MDI (metered dose inhaler): An inhaler that releases a metered or specific dose of medication mist with the assistance of a propellant.

Micronutrient: An essential nutrient such as a trace mineral or vitamin that is required only in minute amounts.

Nonsteroidal: An anti-inflammatory drug that does not contain steroids.

Obstructive lung disease: A disease condition that in some obstructs the ability for regular airflow because of loss of tissue function or integrity, or blockages that impair the passing of airflow.

Oxygenated: The condition of having oxygen present.

Peristalsis: The movement of indigestible material through the intestine.

Phytochemical: A chemical that occurs naturally in a plant, important to health.

Pneumonia: An acute disease in which the air sacs (alveoli) become filled with fluid or congestion. Usually characterized by a fever, cough, or blood-tinged phlegm.

Protein: Organic substance built of amino acids constituting a large requirement in the diet of animals and humans.

Pulmonary: Of the lungs.

Pulmonary rehabilitation: A comprehensive program designed to include a variety of therapies to treat those with chronic lung conditions. Involves addressing psychological, emotional, educational, and physical conditions.

Pursed lip breathing: A method of breathing that prolongs exhalation and builds back pressure in the airways, relieving air trapping and reducing shortness of breath by allowing a greater amount of oxygenated air into the lungs for gas exchange. Performed by shaping lips in a small circular shape upon exhalation.

Rescue breather: A term used for a short acting bronchodilator that is used in emergency situations to relieve wheezing or shortness of breath.

Respiratory: Pertaining to respiration, the respiratory system in mammals, or the lungs.

Restrictive lung disease: One of two types of lung disease. Any diseases that restrict the ability of the lungs to expand or prevent/reduce the ability for gas exchange to take place from the outside of the lung. Examples include skeletal abnormalities or diseases resulting in a thickening of membranes resulting in loss of ability for gas exchange.

Steroidal: Anti-inflammatory that contains steroids.

Tracheobronchitis: Infection resulting in inflammation of the upper airways. Generally a mild, self-limiting disease but may progress in some cases.

APPENDIX: WRITE IT DOWN!
MY TRACKING CHARTS

My Health-Care Providers

PHYSICIAN NAME	ADDRESS	PHONE	SPECIALTY
Example: Dr. Jones	123 Main St.	222-555-1212	Primary care

My Pulmonary Function Test (PFT) Results

TEST	RESULT/ DATE	RESULT/ DATE	RESULT/ DATE	RESULT/ DATE	RESULT/ DATE
Provider/facility	Example: ABC Medical				
Therapist name	Dawn Fielding				
Tidal volume					
Residual volume					
Total lung capacity					
Functional residual capacity					
FEVI					
FEF 25–75					
FEVI/FVC					
PEFR					

My Six Minute Walk Test Results

Name: _____

Date: _____

Age: _____

Time: _____

Initial Assessment   Y/N   Follow-up Assessment   Y/N

Walk 1   Y/N   Walk 2   Y/N   Walk 3   Y/N

Bronchodilator/time since last dose: _____

BP		Oxygen Use		Gait Aid	Max HR: (220-age)
		_____lpm		Y/N	
Time Mins	**SpO2**	**HR**	**BORG 1–10**	**Rest**	
Rest				Y/N	
0:30				Y/N	
1:00				Y/N	
1:30				Y/N	
2:00				Y/N	
2:30				Y/N	
3:00				Y/N	
3:30				Y/N	
4:00				Y/N	
4:30				Y/N	
5:00				Y/N	
5:30				Y/N	
6:00				Y/N	
Recovery 1					
Recovery 2					

Distance: _____

Rests: _____

SOB: _____

Low Spo2: _____

High HR: _____

Additional Notes/Observations: _____

_____

_____

Signature of Practitioner: _____

My Pulmonary Rehab Team

Facility	
Respiratory specialist	
Physical therapist	
Occupational therapist	
Dietician	
Social worker/counselor	

My Pulmonary Rehab Schedule

SUN	MON	TUES	WED	THU	FRI	SAT

My Pharmacies

PHARMACY	PHARMACIST NAME	ADDRESS	PHONE	DRUG

My Symptom Tracking Chart

Chart which symptoms you have personally experienced so you can report them to your physician.

SYMPTOM	Y/N	FREQUENCY	DURATION	TELL DOCTOR
Worsening shortness of breath (dyspnea)				
Mucus production				
Chest tightness				
Increased frequency of flu or colds				
Persistent cough				
Exposure to risk factors (tobacco, occupational dust/chemicals, other smoke, etc.)				

Weight loss							
Muscle weakness							
*Rapid heart rate							
*Inability to "catch your breath" while talking							
*Loss of mental alertness							
*Discoloration of lips							
*Discoloration of nail beds							
*Recommended treatment for symptoms isn't working or symptoms worsen							

*These symptoms require emergency care. You should note them on this chart so you can share all of this information with your doctor.

My Medications

TYPE	NAME	PHYSICIAN	DOSAGE	FREQUENCY/ TIME OF DAY	FOR HOW LONG?	FOR WHAT SYMPTOMS?	SPECIAL INSTRUCTIONS
Bronchodilators							
Antibiotics							
Anti-inflammatory medications							
Combined drug inhalation therapy medications (MDI/DEP/NEB)							

Cough medications														
Mucus-controlling medications														
Anti-infective medications														
Other medications														

My Asthma Rescue Medications

NAME	DOSAGE		

My Monthly Medications: Refill Calendar

SUN	MON	TUES	WED	THU	FRI	SAT

My Monthly Dose Counter

DAY/DATE	MEDICATION NAME	NUMBER OF ACTUATIONS

My Peak Expiratory Flow (PEF) Tracking Sheet

DAY/DATE	TIME OF DAY	MEASUREMENT

My Asthma Action Plan

My Name:
Physician's Name and Number

Medication	Dose	Frequency

Green Zone 80–100% control	Actions
Usual activity, exercise, and other activitie s Usual cough, phlegm, and mucus Sleeping well Appetite is well and eating is normal	Take medicine as recommended Use oxygen as prescribed Continue regular exercise/activity Continue regular diet plan Avoid cigarette smoke/irritants always Other:

Yellow Zone 50–70% control	Actions
More breathless than usual/shortness of breath Less energy/unable to perform usual tasks Increased cough/phlegm and mucus Use of rescue breather necessary Poor sleep/waking up Loss of appetite Medication not as effective as normal Increased wheezing	Take medicine as recommended Use oxygen as prescribed Use rescue breather/2 puffs every 20 min Continue regular diet plan Avoid cigarette smoke/irritants always Call physician to report changes Start oral corticosteroid Start antibiotic Used PLB Call physician if symptoms don't improve Get extra rest Measure/monitor peak flow

Red Zone <50% control	Actions
Severe shortness of breath even at rest Not able to do activities because of breathing Sleep interrupted because of breathing Fever/chills Heaviness in chest/chest pain Coughing up blood/uncontrollable mucus Rescue meds not working Symptoms not improving	Call 911/seek immediate medical help

My COPD Action Plan

My Name:
Physician's Name and Number

Medication	Dose	Frequency

Green Zone 80–100% control	Actions
Usual activity, exercise, and other activitie s Usual cough, phlegm, and mucus Sleeping well Appetite is well and eating is normal	Take medicine as recommended Use oxygen as prescribed Continue regular exercise/activity Continue regular diet plan Avoid cigarette smoke/irritants always Other:

Yellow Zone 50–70% control	Actions
More breathless than usual/shortness of breath Less energy/unable to perform usual tasks Increased cough/phlegm and mucus Use of rescue breather necessary Poor sleep/waking up Loss of appetite Medication not as effective as normal Increased wheezing	Take medicine as recommended Use oxygen as prescribed Use rescue breather _____ times today Continue regular diet plan Avoid cigarette smoke/irritants always Call physician to report changes Start oral corticosteroid Start antibiotic Used PLB Call physician if symptoms don't improve Get extra rest

Red Zone <50% control	Actions
Severe shortness of breath even at rest Not able to do activities because of breathing Sleep interrupted because of breathing Fever/chills Heaviness in chest/chest pain Coughing up blood/uncontrollable mucus Rescue meds not working Symptoms not improving	Call 911/seek immediate medical help

My New Symptoms

DATE	SYMPTOM/CHANGE
Example: 3/15/15	**Headache, sinus pain**

My Asthma Triggers

DATE	POSSIBLE TRIGGER	RESPONSE

My Hypoxemia Symptoms

DATE/TIME	LITER FLOW/ DEVICE	SYMPTOMS	CAUSE	RESOLUTION

My Exacerbation (Flare-Up) Symptoms

	COUGH	MUCUS COLOR	MUCUS CONSISTENCY	WHEEZING	FEVER	CHEST TIGHTNESS	CHANGE MEDS
Date:							
Date:							
Date:							
Date:							

My Asthma Exacerbations

DAY	NIGHT	ACTIVITY	EXPOSURE	EMOTIONS

My Oxygen Use and Activities

ACTIVITY	REQUIRED LITER FLOW (LITERS PER MINUTE)								
Walking									
Cooking									
Cleaning									
Eating									
Resting									
Talking									
Exercising									
Bathing									
Driving									

Caution:

Oxygen in Use

No Smoking

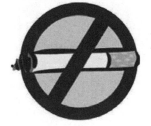

My Oxygen Provider Information

MY OXYGEN PROVIDER	
Name:	
Address:	
Contact Person:	
Concentrator Type:	
Phone: Serial Number:	

My Durable Medical Equipment Provider Information

MY DME EQUIPMENT PROVIDER	
Company Name	
Address:	
Phone:	
Contact Person:	
Phone: Equipment Type:	

My Relaxation Record

DAY	METHOD USED	LENGTH	SUCCESSFUL	TIME OF DAY
Sunday			Y/N	
Monday			Y/N	
Tuesday			Y/N	
Wednesday			Y/N	
Thursday			Y/N	
Friday			Y/N	
Saturday			Y/N	

My Smoking Triggers

List your cravings and what preceded those cravings to help establish what some of your triggers may be.

TIME OF DAY	ACTIVITY PRIOR TO CRAVING

My Quitting Goals

Think about your short-term, medium-term, and advanced goals when it comes to quitting smoking. Write these here to remind yourself to stick to it!

SHORT-TERM GOALS	LONG-TERM GOALS	ADVANCED GOALS

My Quitting Smoking Contract

I,_____, make a promise to myself to quit smoking to improve my life, my own well-being, and the well-being of those I love. I promise to forgive myself for past failed attempts at quitting and approach this occasion with celebration and excitement. I promise to take each day one at a time (and even one hour at a time if I need to) while I wean myself off the nicotine addiction I have. I promise to surround myself with people who support me and want to help. I promise to ask for help if I need it.

I will quit on the_____day of _____, 20_____.

My Signature:_____Date:_____

My Sponsor's Signature: _____Date:_____

Calendar of Days That I Quit

Mark the days as they pass. Be sure to reward yourself when you reach your goals.

SUN	MON	TUES	WED	THU	FRI	SAT

SUPPORTIVE ONLINE RESOURCES

For more information on the COPD Solution program, downloadable worksheets, and other resources, please visit www.thecopdsolution.com.

There are many other valuable resources online; here is a list of the best of them:

COPD RESOURCES

www.aafa.org   www.COPD-International.com
www.asthma.com   www.emphysemafoundation.org
www.chroniclungalliance.org   www.livingwithcopd.com
www.copdfoundation.org

PULMONARY HYPERTENSION RESOURCES

www.americanheart.org   www.phaassociation.org
www.chroniclungalliance.org

CYSTIC FIBROSIS RESOURCES

www.cff.org

FOOD GUIDE PYRAMID

www.108degreehealth.com   www.nourrishedkitchen.com
www.eatwell.com   www.nutrition.gov
www.foodbabe.com   www.theperennialplate.com
www.mypyramid.gov   www.twobluelemons.com

ACCP PATIENT EDUCATION SHEETS FOR INHALER USE

www.chestnet.org/patients/guides/inhaledDevices.php
www.chroniclungalliance.org

ALL LUNG CONDITIONS

American Lung Association: www.lungusa.org
Chronic Lung Alliance: www.chroniclungalliance.org
National Heart, Lung, and Blood Institution: nhlbi.nih.gov

ASTHMA RESOURCES

American Lung Association: www.lung.org
Asthma and Allergy Foundation of America: www.aafa.org
Chronic Lung Alliance: www.chroniclungalliance.org

ABOUT THE AUTHOR

Dawn Lesley Fielding, RCP, AE-C, has a mission and deep passion for the cause of serving people with chronic obstructive pulmonary disease (COPD). A licensed respiratory therapist, certified COPD educator, certified asthma educator, patient advocate, and pulmonary rehab clinical specialist with years of hands-on experience working with people with COPD and managing a pulmonary rehabilitation center, she has firsthand experience with the desperation of breathing distress, as her own son suffers from bad asthma. Dawn also founded the Chronic Lung Alliance, a nonprofit dedicated to educating those who suffer with chronic lung disease and their families, friends, and care providers. www.thecopdsolution.com

INDEX